# MILESTONES IN DANCE HISTORY

This introduction to world dance charts the diverse histories and stories of dancers and artists through ten key moments that have shaped the vast spectrum of different forms and genres that we see today.

Designed for weekly use in dance history courses, ten chosen milestones move chronologically from the earliest indigenous rituals and the dance crazes of Eastern trade routes, to the social justice performance and evolving online platforms of modern times. This clear, dynamic framework uses the idea of migrations to chart the shifting currents of influence and innovation in dance from an inclusive set of perspectives that acknowledge the enduring cultural legacies on display in every dance form.

Milestones are a range of accessible textbooks, breaking down the need-to-know moments in the social, cultural, political, and artistic development of foundational subject areas.

**Dana Tai Soon Burgess** is the Smithsonian Institution's first ever choreographer in residence based at the National Portrait Gallery. He is the artistic director of Washington, DC's premiere modern dance company, Dana Tai Soon Burgess Dance Company, now in its 30th season. He is a professor of dance at The George Washington University and host of The Slant Podcast.

# Milestones Series

Milestones are a range of accessible textbooks, breaking down the need-to-know moments in the social, cultural, political, and artistic development of foundational subject areas. Each book maps out ten key moments in the development of its subject, from the emergence of an academic discipline or the chronology of a period in history, to the evolution of an idea or school of thought.

The Milestones books are ideal for undergraduate students, either as degree primers or classroom textbooks. The ten key moments make them an ideal fit for weekly class reading and easily digestible for individual study.

**Milestones in Dance History**
*edited by Dana Tai Soon Burgess*

**Milestones in Staging Gender and Sexuality**
*edited by Emily Rollie*

**Milestones in Asian American Theatre**
*edited by Josephine Lee*

**Milestones in Black American Theatre and Performance**
*edited by Monica W. Ndounou*

**Milestones in Musical Theatre**
*edited by Mary Jo Lodge*

**Milestones in Dance in the USA**
*edited by Elizabeth McPherson*

For more information about this series, please visit: https://www.routledge.com/Milestones/book-series/MILES

# MILESTONES IN DANCE HISTORY

### Edited by Dana Tai Soon Burgess

Routledge
Taylor & Francis Group

LONDON AND NEW YORK

Cover image: Dana Tai Soon Burgess Dance Company, 2017 by Jeff Watts; and Dana Tai Soon Burgess Dance Company performs *A Tribute to Marian Anderson*, 2019 by Jeff Malet

First published 2023
by Routledge
4 Park Square, Milton Park, Abingdon, Oxon OX14 4RN

and by Routledge
605 Third Avenue, New York, NY 10158

*Routledge is an imprint of the Taylor & Francis Group, an informa business*

*British Library Cataloguing-in-Publication Data*
A catalogue record for this book is available from the British Library

*Library of Congress Cataloging-in-Publication Data*
Names: Burgess, Dana Tai Soon, editor.
Title: Milestones in dance history / edited by Dana Tai Soon Burgess.
Description: Abingdon, Oxon; New York, NY: Routledge, 2023. |
Series: Milestones | Includes bibliographical references and index.
Identifiers: LCCN 2022008982 (print) | LCCN 2022008983 (ebook) |
ISBN 9781032029405 (paperback) | ISBN 9781032029412 (hardback) |
ISBN 9781003185918 (ebook)
Subjects: LCSH: Dance—History.
Classification: LCC GV1601 ,M55 2023 (print) | LCC GV1601 (ebook) |
DDC 793.3/19—dc23/eng/20220519
LC record available at https://lccn.loc.gov/2022008982
LC ebook record available at https://lccn.loc.gov/2022008983

ISBN: 978-1-032-02941-2 (hbk)
ISBN: 978-1-032-02940-5 (pbk)
ISBN: 978-1-003-18591-8 (ebk)

DOI: 10.4324/9781003185918

Typeset in Bembo and Scala Sans
by codeMantra

In memory of my father, Joseph James Burgess, Jr. (1924–2014), who taught me to love learning

# Contents

Contents

# Contributors

Kathryn Boland

Joanna Dee Das

Monique George

Laurel Victoria Gray

Kate Mattingly

Maria Francisca Morand

Sekani Robinson

Giselle Ruzany

Dana Tai Soon Burgess

Tria Blu Wakpa

# Foreword

*Dana Tai Soon Burgess*

Throughout the world, people dance. Movement is a universal language with the capacity to communicate beyond borders and to build bridges of understanding that span socio-economic, political, and cultural divides. *Milestones in Dance History* is a fresh framework for teaching dance history that allows the reader to make global dance connections between antiquity and modernity. The book illuminates the relationship of dance stories to key historical events, including the forced migrations of slavery from West Africa to the Americas, the exchange of culture and commerce along the ancient trade routes of the Silk Road, artistic shifts that accompanied changes in political and social mores during the interwar period between WWI and WWII, and the evolution of the interactive relationship between dance and technology.

*Milestones in Dance History* refocuses the canon of dance history by contextualizing it with watershed moments of migration and political conflict, as well as with personal stories and those of cultural icons that have shaped the artform. The authors are notable dance artists, practitioners, and scholars, from varying cultural backgrounds, who write through lenses of inclusivity. *Milestones in Dance History* celebrates dance by presenting episodes that chronicle the dances of distinct cultures, the work of acclaimed dancers, choreographers and film directors, the rise of dance technology, and the impact of shifting geopolitical landscapes on the art and lives of dancers. This book is especially timely as societies around the world reconsider their cultural legacies and seek to decolonize the canon of dance.

*Milestones in Dance History* is divided into ten chronologically based chapters; each focuses on key landmark moments in dance. These include the continued evolution and resiliency of indigenous dances as tribal solidarity and protest at Standing Rock, the migration of dances in ancient times and modern day along the famed Silk Road trade route that connects the East and West, and the forced migrations of dances due to slavery from West Africa to the Americas that shaped the vernacular of American dance. The chapter on ballet traces the history of racialized casting and segregation on stage which is finally moving to inclusivity. The development of modern dance and the field of dance as healing are contextualized by major political shifts between WWI and WWII which displaced artists and changed and challenged their aesthetics. Social justice is exemplified by the contemporary embodiment of the historic repertoire of the first Asian-American modern dance choreographer whose career was nearly erased by an Executive Order. Changing dance aesthetics due to the evolution of technological advancements, including the film industry in Los Angeles and Mumbai, are discussed in relation to the life episodes of acclaimed dancers, choreographers, and film directors. The history of dance and Artificial Intelligence (AI) interactivity is traced back to theatrical flying machinery and, finally, a stimulating projection of the future of dance poses the question of what dancing in the new frontiers of space might entail.

I hope *Milestones in Dance History* will inspire young dancers, future choreographers, and dance scholars, as well as audience members, to make dance connections across the globe and between various time periods. After reading *Milestones in Dance History*, I believe you will want to delve deeper into the stories that make up dance history and explore the *Further Readings* list at the end of the book. As we uncover and acknowledge, both the celebratory, as well as the painfully flawed parts of our history, we can engage in deeper conversations that lead us to a better understanding of the universal language of dance.

# Acknowledgments

Claire-Solène Bečka
Kristina Berger
Kathryn Boland
Joanna Dee Das
Zoë Forbes
Jameson Freeman
Monique George
Laurel Victoria Gray
Steph Hines
Deborah Hofmann-Asimov
Michael Kaiser
Kate Mattingly
Maria Francisca Morand
Ben Piggott
Sekani Robinson
Giselle Ruzany
Tria Blu Wakpa

# CHAPTER 1

# Indigenous Dances
## Lakota Bodies and Lands on and as the Frontlines

*Tria Blu Wakpa*

The creative possibilities of movement modes – such as writing[1] and dance – can critically counter the ways that U.S. **settler colonialism** and capitalism subordinate Indigenous peoples and people of color.[2] As Audre Lorde – a "Black, lesbian, mother, warrior, poet"[3] – articulates:

> poetry is not a luxury. It is a vital necessity of our existence. It forms the quality of the light within which we predicate our hopes and dreams toward survival and change, first made into language, then into idea, then into more tangible action.

For Native Americans whom the U.S. has often attempted to annihilate and assimilate, Indigenous dance may similarly be viewed as "not a luxury."[4] U.S. colonizers have policed, prohibited, appropriated, leveraged, and (mis)represented Native dance for settler colonial and capitalist purposes. Meanwhile, many Indigenous peoples have continued to dance to enact dreams, prayer, storytelling, **sovereignty**, solidarity, social change, and survival. The enduring, interlocking, and anthropocentric structures of settler colonialism and capitalism frequently prioritize profit over the wellbeing of humans and our more-than-human kin, such as nonhuman animals, air, land, water, and the cosmos with whom people are inextricably linked.[5] Unjustly dispossessed of their lands, but often continuing to recognize, and when possible, enact relationships with these lands, Native peoples by their very presence undermine the legitimacy and authority of the U.S., including its claims to democracy, egalitarianism, and

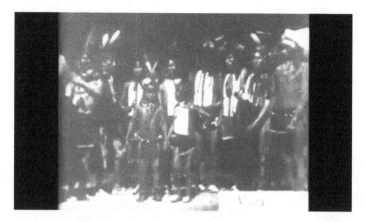

**Figure 1.1:** Seven Up, the boy standing center and stage left, momentarily looks towards one of the men, perhaps for reassurance. Still from Dickson, *Sioux Ghost Dance* (0:09).
Source: Retrieved from Library of Congress, www.loc.gov/item/00694139/.
Author's screenshot. Library of Congress, Motion Picture, Broadcasting, and Recorded Sound Division.

freedom. This chapter delineates how Indigenous dances can combat what Shannon Speed refers to as "settler capitalist power"[6] and nurture and protect relationships with more-than-humans.

To combat settler colonial "histories" that frequently obscure Indigenous peoples and practices as well as relegate them to the past, this chapter centers a constellation of Native dance films, from 1894 to 2016, related to Lakota bodies and lands that demonstrate how Indigenous dancers have adapted and innovated their movement modes, which have circulated widely via the cutting-edge technology of their times and continue to do so today. In both the past and present, the U.S. and international imaginary tend to center Lakota people, practices, lands, and forms of resistance; yet, these narratives often overlook the knowledge that Lakota and other Indigenous peoples express through movement modes on Lakota lands. All of the films that I analyze, from the **Kinetoscope** to social media, are one-shot shorts currently available open-access on YouTube and Facebook. In contrast to live performances, dance films can provide an archive that allows new viewers who were not present for the original presentation to examine the movement qualities, knowledges, and critiques offered, providing powerful insights into how Native peoples and practices have survived and adapted. Given U.S. assimilation policies, including nearly a century of prohibitions surrounding Indigenous dances and spiritualities,[7] Indigenous peoples today may also draw on archival documents such as films for the purposes of cultural revitalization.[8] In conversation with Audre Lorde's "Poetry Is Not a Luxury," which highlights the interconnections among poetry, dreams, political action, and survival – I delineate how these Indigenous dances articulate timely and powerful challenges to settler colonial structures and discourses by enacting alternative imaginings that are often excluded from mainstream and scholarly discourses. Given the ways that settler colonial narratives operate, the visibility of Indigenous peoples, practices, and issues – including through Indigenous dance films – may be a vital first step towards justice, and viewing dance in particular creates what Susan Foster terms "kinesthetic empathy,"[9] which can inspire and compel social change.

This chapter emphasizes the endurance of Indigenous dancing on and *as* the *frontlines*, a fraught and enduring frontier space, which I conceptualize broadly in and beyond the specific geographies typically associated with social movements to demonstrate how settler-capitalism is pervasive and entrenched in U.S. society. Because through their very presence, Indigenous peoples interfere with the aim of settler colonialism – which is for settlers to make their home on Native lands[10] – their very bodies and movement modes can be conceived of as the "frontlines." This illustrates not only how the "frontlines" can be embodied, but also the inextricable linkages between Indigenous bodies and lands. Such an expansive understanding of "frontlines" further challenges myths that settler colonialism is settled – that is, Indigenous lands, which compose the entirety of what is often referred to as the U.S., are no longer contested – and Native peoples and practices are static and relegated to a historic past and, in particular, often rural and/or peripheral locales.[11] The applicability of Lorde's words from a Black feminist perspective to

Indigenous contexts demonstrates how cultural productions depicting movement modalities can be critical for subaltern peoples' survival. Also highlighting the commonalities among diverse Black and Native experiences, in 2021, U.S. poet laureate, Joy Harjo (Mvskoke Nation) named Lorde's writings on survival as vital to Harjo's own "survival book" of poetry.[12] This gestures to the linkages between Black liberation and Indigenous sovereignty, which are apparent on the frontlines.[13] These interconnections occur because U.S. settler colonial structures have often operated to manage the bodies and movements of Black peoples and Indigenous peoples and more-than-humans in ways that infringe on their freedom and futurities, what I have termed "settler colonial choreographies."[14]

Colonizers have frequently sought to construct Indigenous dances as a marker of difference, through attempts to hierarchize non-Natives above Native peoples by associating Eurocentric peoples and practices with progress and the future and their Indigenous counterparts with primitivity and the past.[15] Yet, all dances change every time they are enacted because exact repetition of an embodied act is impossible,[16] and "traditional" Native dances can and are choreographed in contemporary times. When applied to Native peoples and practices, concepts of Indigenous dances as "authentic" or "traditional" can also operate as an attempt to "measure" their "Indianness," a settler colonial strategy that works to undermine Native peoples' "authenticity" – specifically their unique status as citizens of, and/or connection to Native nations and lands.[17]

The Indigenous dances I analyze are inextricably intertwined with Indigenous visions, spirituality, storytelling, corporeal and social movements, and **survivance**; in this way, they can be read as staunch critiques of ongoing colonization within settler colonial constraints. First, I contextualize why this chapter focuses on Lakota people and lands. Then, in order to show how the "frontlines" has been a central feature of Native dance films since their origins, I conduct close readings of bodies, corporeal and social movements, and articles and/or interviews in regard to the 1894 film

*Sioux Ghost Dance* – one of the first to depict Native people onscreen – as well as contemporary online films of Jingle Dress Dancing and a traditional Māori dancer, Kereama Te Ua, offering the haka in support of the 2016–2017 movement to stop the Dakota Access Pipeline. Lakota activist and attorney Chase Iron Eyes has called the 2016–2017 #NoDAPL movement "our Ghost Dance."[18] Although settler colonial narratives often relegate the Ghost Dance – a pan-Indigenous movement "practiced among many groups from the plains to California in the 1880s"[19] – to the past, as Iron Eyes articulates, its aims endure and innovate today.[20]

Charting a constellation of Lakota dances and lands on the frontlines from "*Ghost Dance*" to "Ghost Dance" – that is 1894 to 2016 – I depart from settler colonial, linear histories, with their presumptions of U.S. progress and Native extinction.[21] My purpose in this chapter is to provide the vital historical, political, and cultural contexts that motivate and underpin these dances, which is necessary for viewers to understand these movement modes and the ongoing struggles that Indigenous peoples endure globally, including how Indigenous "histories" and contemporary circumstances may interweave. Māori peoples, like Native Americans, have also endured, negotiated, and resisted the violence of colonization, including attacks on their dances and Indigenous more-than-humans.[22] Each of the Indigenous dances I analyze can be read in ways that combat and critique settler colonialism while making visible Native epistemologies and imaginings through vivid bodily expressions.

## THE LAKOTA CONTEXT

Lakota people have often been at the forefront of Indigenous resistance to settler colonialism and a target for U.S. prohibitions, punishments, and violence surrounding Indigenous dances. They are indigenous to the lands from what is often called "northern Colorado to central North Dakota [and] from central Wyoming to eastern South Dakota" in the partition of Turtle Island frequently referred to as the U.S.[23]

In the 1876 Battle of Greasy Grass, Lakota people, along with the Northern Cheyenne and Arapaho, defeated the 7th Cavalry Regiment.[24] From the 1800s to the 1978 American Indian Religious Freedom Act, the U.S. government outlawed some Native dances.[25] Jacqueline Shea Murphy writes that U.S. colonizers viewed "Indian dancing as barbaric and immoral," and in particular, targeted the Sun Dance, a ceremony of the Lakota and other Plains Indian peoples.[26] Although narratives often attribute Lakota interest in the Ghost Dance to Wovoka, a Paiute man, the movement is frequently associated with Lakota people and the subsequent 1890 Wounded Knee Massacre in which the 7th Cavalry Regiment murdered 300 Lakota people, the majority of whom were children, women, and elders.[27]

Via the interconnected realms of entertainment and activism, Lakota people, dances, and lands have also been significant in shaping both the U.S. and international imagination in regard to Native Americans from the late 19th century to the present day. As Harald E.L. Prins notes,

> given their long experience with mythistory, blurring fact and fiction, it is not surprising to see indigenous activists move back and forth between the real and reel. Continuing a performance tradition stretching back to Sitting Bull and Black Elk in the 1880s, and even before, some of [the American Indian Movement's] most visible leaders have accepted prominent Hollywood roles.[28]

Despite U.S. prohibitions of Indigenous dances, Indigenous people danced in secret as well as in public settings – such as Wild West shows, which were many times non-Native run endeavors.[29] Although banning Indigenous dance in private settings and encouraging it in the public sphere may seem contradictory, both strategies are congruent with "settler-capitalist"[30] structures. Buffalo Bill's Wild West show, which traveled throughout the U.S., Canada, and Europe, often recruited Lakota people to be the Native performers.[31] Following the Wounded Knee Massacre, Buffalo Bill Cody hired Lakota people who were imprisoned for Ghost Dancing *to dance* in his shows, advertising the Lakota actors and their dances as "authentic."[32] In addition to offering freedom from incarceration, some Lakota people viewed acting in Wild West shows as an opportunity to earn a living, perpetuate and innovate their lifeways, and travel.[33]

In the 20th and 21st centuries, Lakota people have continued to contest and negotiate settler colonial structures and discourses while contributing to social change in critical ways. In the 1960s and 1970s, Lakota people served as leaders in Native activist endeavors, including the initial 1964 Alcatraz Occupation, the 1972 "Trail of Broken Treaties" march to Washington, D.C. and subsequent occupation of the Bureau of Indian Affairs, and the 1973 Wounded Knee Occupation.[34] The 1973 Wounded Knee Occupation was also referred to by some as a "Ghost Dance."[35] Some Lakota people participated in the inaugural 1978 Longest Walk, a peaceful and spiritual, 3000-mile journey from Alcatraz Island to Washington, D.C.[36] The Longest Walk brought attention to Native peoples and issues and resulted in the passage of the 1978 American Indian Religious Freedom Act, evidencing how peaceful protest through movement modes has resulted in significant social change.[37]

Cultural productions by and about Lakota people and Lakota-led social movements have also garnered mainstream attention in the 1990s and into the present day. In 1990, Mary Brave Bird published her memoir *Lakota Woman*, a national best seller and winner of the American Book Award.[38] *Dances with Wolves*, the "epic," Hollywood Western film, which grossed $424 million worldwide, was shot on Lakota lands and also released in 1990.[39] Notably, the film, which has been critiqued as reifying settler colonial narratives, has the word "dances" in the title, again a practice that has been leveraged to signify Native difference.[40] Most recently, in 2016–2017, Lakota and Dakota people on Lakota and Dakota lands led "the largest Native American protest movement in living memory" in opposition to the Dakota Access pipeline, which mainstream media outlets covered at least in part.[41] At the time, Lakota activist and attorney Chase Iron Eyes referred to this movement as "our Ghost Dance," evidencing the through lines of the frontlines, ongoing colonization, Indigenous resistance, and the inextricable linkages between Native movement modes, in this case, Indigenous dance and Native social movements.[42]

## Sioux Ghost Dance

The 1894 film *Sioux Ghost Dance*, shot in Thomas Edison's Black Maria Studio, shows not only how non-Native people and institutions from the late 19th century until today have (mis)represented Lakota dances for settler-capitalist purposes, but also offers insight into how Lakota people have navigated and thwarted these impositions.[43] *Sioux Ghost Dance* is a 20 second, black and white, single-shot, silent film.[44] It features 11 Oglala and Brule Lakota men and boys, although 15 Lakota actors were purportedly present that day: Chief Last Horse, Parts His Hair, Black Cat, Hair Coat, Charging Crow, Dull Knife, Holy Bear, Crazy Bear, Strong Talker, Pine, Little Eagle, Young Bear, Runs Above, Johnny Burke No Neck, and Seven Up.[45] On September 24, 1894, the Lakota actors, along with Buffalo Bill Cody, traveled by train to West Orange, New Jersey, where the Black Maria Studio was located.[46] At the time, Buffalo Bill's Wild West show was holding performances nearby in Brooklyn's Ambrose Park.[47] William Kennedy-Laurie Dickson directed *Sioux Ghost Dance* while William Heise "manned the kinetograph, the camera that shot film for the [peephole] kinetoscope."[48] According to scholar Michael Gaudio,

> A customer would pay twenty-five cents to see five films or fifty cents for all ten and then peer into a kinetoscope's peephole and watch for about twenty seconds as fifty feet of film sped by on a continuous spool.... [B]y the end of [1894], kinetoscope parlors...[existed] across the country from Boston to San Francisco.[49]

Although the esteemed Oglala Lakota leader Crazy Horse[50] – who was born in approximately 1840 and died in 1877 – famously said that he did not want his photograph taken because it might "capture his spirit," clearly Lakota people have had diverse responses to their representation in media.[51]

The 1894 films of the Wild West show performers provided exciting material for Kinetoscope viewers, mostly described in scholarship as White audiences, which was not separate from the racialization of Native peoples.[52] Similar to Jacqueline Shea Murphy's argument that Native American dance is emblematic of Native and non-Native difference, Gaudio writes, "The fact that two of the four films made that day were dances from the Wild West show suggests that...the subject of Native American dance remained a powerful one for audiences to satisfy their curiosity for strange peoples and customs through lifelike images."[53] This description notably centers the reactions of White viewers. The creation of the films also illustrates the settler colonial impulse towards "salvage ethnography" or the documentation of "authentic" Native practices before they shift or become extinct.[54] Again, this is problematic because all dances change every time they are performed, and although settler colonial narratives frequently portray Native peoples, dances, and languages as naturally endangered or dying out, it is U.S. practices, policies, and prohibitions that have detrimentally impacted them.[55]

Evidencing the historic and enduring settler-capitalist (mis) representation of Lakota dance, *Sioux Ghost Dance* actually depicts an Omaha Dance, advertised as a "war dance" in Wild West shows.[56] "Sioux" is also an outsider term for the Lakota, Dakota, and Nakota peoples, and many view it as less preferable to their names for themselves and even see it as derogatory.[57] In contrast, newspaper articles about the filming from 1894 refer to the dance as an "Omaha war dance," which is still not quite correct and privileges a settler-capitalist lens.[58] Although the dance was/is related to "warfare protection" and can reenact "warfare achievements and victories," Lakota experts typically refer/referred to it as an "Omaha dance."[59] As evidenced in Ben Black Bear, Sr. and R.D. Theisz's *Songs and Dances of the Lakota People*, some Lakota-centered descriptions of the "Omaha dance" do not even mention the word "war."[60] Gaudio also notes that the film might have circulated under the name of *Sioux Ghost Dance* in the 1890s.[61] Like the name "Omaha war dance," the title *Sioux Ghost Dance* likely operated as a form of advertisement, as many viewers at the time would have been aware of the Wounded Knee Massacre, frequently and problematically portrayed in settler discourses as a "battle."[62] Today, the Library of Congress website, relying on a description from Edison films catalog, continues to provide misleading information about the film: "One of the most peculiar customs of the Sioux Tribe is shown here, the dancers being genuine Sioux Indians, in full-war paint and war costumes."[63] This representation problematically portrays the Omaha dance as "peculiar," and the actors as "genuine" or "authentically" Native, a strategy, as I have discussed, that Buffalo Bill Cody used to advertise his shows.[64] The description also does not provide any indication that the title of the film is *not* the type of dance being depicted. However, as Gaudio writes, drawing on movement descriptions of Ghost Dancing, which significantly contrast with the Omaha Dance seen in the film, "Any viewer who has basic familiarity with the Ghost Dance can easily see that this is not the dance we witness."[65] The Library of Congress further uses the keyword "Dakota" in regard to *Sioux Ghost Dance*; however, the dancers are Lakota.[66] Many Native people also prefer not to use the term "costume" to refer to the regalia they wear for spiritual purposes.[67]

Although *Sioux Ghost Dance* can and certainly has been interpreted in ways that reify settler colonial tropes of Native peoples and practices, I am interested in a counter reading that reveals how the Lakota dancers combat and critique these stereotypes. The politics of the Omaha dance and the dancers' identities indeed encourage such an analysis. As Mark G. Thiel writes, "For generations, the Omaha dance has been the most popular social and nationalistic celebration of the Oglala Sioux and Sicangu Sioux, thus serving as an obtrusive demonstration of tribal identity and cohesion."[68] In other words, the dance itself challenges settler assumptions about Native domination and assimilation, as do the dancers' identities and regalia. Gaudio highlights that at the time of the Wounded Knee Massacre, the dancers would have been on Lakota lands, in the vicinity of where the horrific act occurred; yet, as this film shows, they continued to dance in Indigenous ways.[69] This evidences how the "frontlines" can be conceptualized not only as a particular place, but also in relation to people, movement modes, and cinematic spaces, which historically and contemporarily have been dominated by non-Native people.[70] Also, a boy who stars in *Sioux Ghost Dance*, Johnny Burke No Neck, was purportedly the only child who survived the Massacre; in this way, he literally embodies those frontlines in the film, which was shot in Brooklyn on Lenape lands, another frontline for Lenape people.[71]

The film opens with Johnny Burke No Neck and another Lakota boy, Seven Up, center stage, surrounded by nine Lakota men; together, they appear to form a frontline facing the camera.[72] The intergenerational group, all clothed in Lakota regalia, challenges the settler myths of Native extinction. Enveloped in moccasins, the boys' feet step to the rhythm of the drum before the adult dancers' do. Along with the moccasins, dancing to the beat of the drum (which is not evident on-screen) represents human connection to mother earth, which can challenge settler-capitalist logics.[73] The dancers' abrupt head movements – resembling that of chickens, prairie chickens, or other birds who are indigenous to Lakota lands – and the eagle and perhaps other more-than-human feathers that they wear also evidence human and more-than-human linkages.[74] Seven Up, his face in profile to the viewer, momentarily looks towards one of the men, perhaps for reassurance. While settler discourses often represent Native men as symbols of resistance, this suggests their roles as father figures.[75] A man, standing on stage left raises and lowers what seems to be a dance stick, at which point the boy turns his face to the earth, hunches his shoulders forward and begins to stomp with an authority and decisiveness, which could be interpreted as a form of self-determination despite power differentials between the Lakota boy and European filmmakers in the studio space.[76] Johnny Burke No Neck opens his mouth, likely to let out an audible sound.[77] He wears two eagle feathers extending from the top of his head while other adult dancers wear one or two eagle feathers. This is notable because as Leo Killsback writes, "[w]arriors who participated in the sun dance ceremony placed a single eagle plume at the top of an extension, protruding upright from the center of the head, signifying their status attained from ceremony."[78] In other words, at a time when U.S. officials were in some instances outlawing Sun Dance and the regalia that accompanied it, Lakota boys and men were flaunting their Lakota identities, practices, rank, and courage for massive audiences.[79]

Connoting the connections among action, dance, spirituality, dreams, and survival, from stage left, the sole Lakota man wearing a war bonnet skillfully glides across the set while keeping rhythm with the drum. A war bonnet may indicate a person is a seasoned and skilled warrior "prepared to die" and reflect "a deliberate [choice] to make himself conspicuous to the enemy just to show how brave he was."[80] Thus, the dancer's centering of himself may have corresponded with his dedication to and distinction in the community, mindset, and boldness. Because "wearers of warbonnets invested a high degree of spirituality to their headdress" and "war bonnets were conceived from dreams or visions made for those seeking protection or personal power," his regalia demonstrates how spirituality and dreams are also inextricable from this Omaha dance.[81] Via the war bonnet, fashioned from feathers, the dance is also interconnected to more-than-humans and Lakota sovereignty and futurity. Killsback explains that the war bonnet "tells of a time when our young men maintained a sacred life of discipline and honor; when men submitted to discipline, loyalty, and sacrifice for the livelihood of their people, land, and future generations."[82] Once the man reaches stage right, this dancer turns a tight circle, momentarily swaggers towards the camera, and then to his left, towards another performer. The two dancers' gazes appear to be locked, inches apart. At this point, they also briefly circle each other while standing nearly upright, although more frequently, they move in a crouched stance with their knees bent. Together, the two performers' gazes and standing positions are perhaps indicative of masculinity and confrontation, evidencing enduring Lakota warrior prowess. Although representations of Lakota men as warriors can reinforce settler colonial stereotypes of Indigenous men as violent, in some Native constructions of masculinity, "the warrior ideal" may describe those who "fight to defend their homes and their cultural communities" which can be both honorable and vital for Indigenous human and more-than-human survival.[83]

Challenging settler colonial constructions of Native people as a monolith, neither the regalia nor the choreography are uniform.[84] Some of the dancers make circles within the collective circle; most step clockwise while others move counterclockwise; at the end of the film, one boy weaves through the circle towards the camera and to stage left.[85] Throughout the majority of the dance, the men envelop the boys, also an embodiment of Lakota futurity, which symbolizes the adults' protectiveness of the youth. Countering misinformed, settler assumptions that Native practices are static and unchanged, the Lakota dancers likely had to adapt their dancing for the limited studio space since they were used to performing outdoors in spacious arenas and community settings.[86] Although the proximity of bodies in the confined space could be read as conveying U.S. containment of Lakota peoples and practices, conversely, the dancers' competent maneuvering illustrates their expertise at navigating settler constraints, literally and figuratively, while contributing to Lakota futures as embodied by the Lakota boys and documented for subsequent circulation by the Kinetograph. Futurity was likely on at least some of the dancers' minds, as an 1894 article titled "Buffalo Bill's Indians Exhibit for the Wonderful Kinetoscope," states that the Lakota dancers "had been told that the strange thing pointed at them…would show them to the world until after the sun had slept his last sleep."[87] The subtitle of this 1894 article states, "FUTURE GENERATIONS TO SEE," and indeed they do in the contemporary day.

## JINGLE DRESS DANCE AT STANDING ROCK

Although over a century separates *Sioux Ghost Dance* and the Jingle Dress Dance on the frontlines at the Standing Rock Indian Reservation, they both illuminate how Native people continue to dance as a survival tactic within U.S.

settler-capitalist society. The Jingle Dress Dance Ceremony occurred on October 29, 2016, two days after an October 27 raid on the Treaty Camp, which was "one of several camps...established to prevent construction of Energy Transfer Partners' $3.8 billion Dakota Access Pipeline (DAPL)."[88] Writing about this raid, Aileen Brown, Will Parrish, and Alice Speri state, "[H]undreds of law enforcement officers descended on a small resistance camp that stood directly in front of the Dakota Access Pipeline, forcibly evicting residents and arresting 142 people – more than on any other day of the 11-month-long Standing Rock."[89] The pipeline crossed two rivers and four states and ran alongside "culturally sensitive sites," but also, as Nick Estes emphasizes, the "No Dakota Pipeline" or NoDAPL movement was "a struggle over the land and water in which a people were fighting for their lives."[90] During the October 27 raid on the Treaty Camp, "law enforcement...deploy[ed] pepper spray, Tasers, rubber bullets, sound cannons, and batons against water protectors."[91] On October 28, 2016, the day following this raid, an elder and Jingle Dress Dancer issued a call for solidarity, for Jingle Dress Dancers "to once again bring our healing dance to the people."[92]

Native movement modes, such as the Jingle Dress Dance, can counter settler-capitalism by offering healing and medicine through **holistic** prayer, which can sustain Native peoples' resistance and survival. According to scholar Mark Thiel, although:

> Many different oral traditions surround the origins of the modern Jingle Dress Dance[,]... Most traditions have similar themes describing the dress as a prayer or medicine dress for healing afflicted people, that came in a dream from spirits or the Creator.[93]

Reminiscent of Audre Lorde's words, dreams inspire the Jingle Dress Dance, as they did Wovoka's Ghost Dance. In these contexts, Native dance, like poetry, "is not a luxury. It is a vital necessity of [Native peoples'] existence. It forms the quality of the light within which [Native people] predicate [their] hopes and dreams toward survival and change."[94]

As Thiel writes, in some cases Jingle Dress Dancers "danced to special songs that re-enacted dreams."[95] Thiel also traces the origins of the Jingle Dress Dance to contexts when survival was often uncertain: World War I and the 1918 influenza pandemic.[96] In some circumstances, people had dreams about the Jingle Dress Dance, which included "songs, a dance, and protocols as a healing prayer," and the ceremony became recognized for its power to cure those who were ill.[97]

The interconnected relationship between humans and more-than-human kin, which was at the heart of the NoDAPL movement, is also apparent in the Jingle Dress Dance.[98] As Tara Browner writes, "In the Jingle Dance, one foot is never to leave the ground, so the dancer always remains connected to the earth."[99] Also evidencing human and more-than-human interconnections, Acosia Red Elk, a ten-time Jingle Dress Dance champion, shared with me a less well-known origin story about the dance, which the elders at Red Lake Nation gifted to her.[100] In this story, the Jingle Dress Dance was a "gift from the Northern Lights" to a man who was in a coma.[101]

> The Northern Light Spirit Beings shared a lot of teachings about the future with him and a lot of information about what was going to happen in the future, and that the people were going to need a message of healing. And that there would be time of separation and that people would begin to separate from one another, and that Nations would be separating from one another, and that people would become separate from their own spirit and from the land.[102]

Notably, people viewing themselves as separate from the land and water is a settler-capitalist logic that allows for the construction of pipelines. Red Elk also explained that the sound the cones on the dress create during the Jingle Dress Dance is

> the vibration and the frequency and the sound that the Northern Lights can make themselves. And it's a

healing vibration, it's a healing sound. That's the sound that a whole bunch of jingle dresses make together, and it's the sound of electricity.[103]

Putting Red Elk's words in conversation with Lorde's, the dream that the man has while in a coma creates the sound, which creates the healing, which creates "survival and change," all of which is inextricable from more-than-humans, in this case, the Northern Lights. This healing sound contrasts strikingly with the sound of cannons that law enforcement at Standing Rock employed to injure water protectors.[104]

In the videos of the Jingle Dress Dance Ceremony on the frontlines at the Standing Rock Indian Reservation, along with drumming and singing, the sounds of the cones are audible and remarkable. Although the filming of ceremonies at Standing Rock camp was typically prohibited, Erin Tapahe, who posted a video of the ceremony on Facebook, wrote, "The dancers invited the media to record it because they want the healing power to be shared with the world."[105] To date, this film has 53,000 reactions and 4,100 comments, indicating how the ceremony's healing power has circulated.[106] The video depicts approximately 30 Native women and girls on an overcast day wearing vividly colorful regalia, together a rainbow of hues, and dancing in a circle on Highway 1806. The dancers are surrounded by people who seem to be their supporters.[107] However, according to writer Simon Moya-Smith, during the ceremony, "Police sat in armored vehicles 150 yards away," evidencing enduring settler state surveillance and tensions on the frontlines.[108] Tonia Jo Hall was one of the Jingle Dress Dancers on the frontlines whose aunt was previously arrested during the raid. Hall shared in a video that she made documenting the experience that she was concerned about her own wellbeing given the violence that the water protectors had recently endured.[109]

While enacting human and more-than-human interconnections through movement, stories, and sound, the Jingle Dress Dance Ceremony at Standing Rock provided an opportunity for water protectors to heal from the violence that they were enduring, which may have been critical to sustaining their peaceful resistance. As Hall explained in a video:

> We need to keep this positive, good feelings and good thoughts. That's what these ceremonies are. Why we brought those ceremonies here... is for those feelings to come back.... With negative, you want to respond with negative, and that's what the DAPL people and the workers want us to respond like. They're trying everything in their power for our people to respond and to retaliate.[110]

Hall's words demonstrate how Native people adapt ceremonies for their contemporary needs, survival tactics, and social action. She also shared,

> Our people went right back to prayer [after the raid] despite rubber bullets, mace, despite beatings with batons, being jerked out of sweat [lodge ceremony]. Our people did exactly what we wanted them to. They went back into prayer. They thought of two ceremonies [the Jingle Dress Dance and the Pipe Ceremonies] that we could have today, and they had those.[111]

Other Indigenous peoples also innovated their dances for Standing Rock amid imminent danger from the settler state.

## HAKA AT STANDING ROCK

The linkages among spirituality, dreams, dances, storytelling, and survival are also evident in the Māori context. The Māori are the Indigenous people of Aotearoa, what is often called New Zealand. Conducting a comparative analysis of the Māori and Lakota peoples from 1840–1920, scholar James Gump discusses how both groups endured "military conquest," "forced acculturation," and land theft.[112] When Gump writes about "[t]he era of contested frontier zones involving the Māori and the Lakota Sioux [which] encompassed a series of treaties and wars that defined relations between these societies and their Western adversaries," he relegates these conflicts to the past; however, the NoDAPL movement illuminates how these struggles continue in the contemporary day.[113] As Nick Estes highlights, DAPL in part "cut through unceded territory of the 1868 Fort Laramie Treaty," which is one reason it was contested.

The Māori and Lakota also similarly responded to colonization by maintaining their Indigenous identities and "turn[ing] to cultural revitalization movements."[114] Gump draws parallels between Ghost Dance in the Lakota context and the Pai Mārire – the "Good and Peaceful" prophecy – which "originated in 1862 from the teachings of Te Ua Haumēne [a Māori prophet] in southern Taranaki."[115] Both movements centered Indigenous visions, included Indigenous dance, and had Christian influences.[116] Although haka is often translated as dance, it is a complex form that has a variety of meanings and purposes, which include storytelling.[117] In the Māori and Lakota contexts, colonizers viewed the Ghost Dance and Pai Mārire suspiciously and killed Indigenous people who were directly or indirectly involved in these practices.[118] Like Native dances on Turtle Island, haka has signified Indigenous and non-Indigenous difference.[119] Colonizers have also appropriated, leveraged, and (mis)represented haka for nationalist and capitalist purposes.[120] Interestingly, dominant culture often misidentifies the haka as a war dance, which is similar to how settler discourses may oversimplify the Omaha Dance.[121] I posit that linking Indigenous men's dances with war – and its connotations of brutality – can be a stereotype that serves colonizers' purposes by attempting to justify settler state intervention, violence, and injustice towards Indigenous peoples. Meanwhile, through the haka, Māori people have enacted sovereignty, solidarity, social change, and survival.[122]

On November 29, 2016, Kereama Te Ua, Māori, did a haka on Lakota lands, on the frontlines of the NoDAPL movement, bringing together the through lines of Lakota and Māori colonization, resistance, and resilience. The haka also illuminates human and more-than-human interdependencies. Te Ua shared with me that the anthem for the

NoDAPL movement, "Mni Wiconi" (Water is Life), also resonated with him and other Māori people who respect water as vital to survival and may even view the more-than-human as an ancestor.[123] Similar to the call that the elder and Jingle Dress Dancer issued, Te Ua shared with me that, even prior to when he traveled to Standing Rock, there was a call for Māori to support the NoDAPL movement by doing the haka collectively at a specified time throughout Aotearoa.[124] This call came from a Facebook group started in Aotearoa titled, "Haka for Standing Rock." Te Ua, along with "hundreds of hundreds of [his] people,"

> went out to the lakes, out to the rivers, out to the ocean, to whichever part of the country they were in, and they sent haka to [the people participating in the NoDAPL movement and their ancestors] through the waterways. They sent them through our rivers and our lakes, through our ocean, sent it up to the heavens. They sent it up through our gods and to support [the ancestors of Turtle Island].[125] He said:

> I can't speak on behalf of those groups or those other tribes, but we all felt that connection...That connection that we have it's our connection to our environment, what we descend from. Our environment is our mother and our father. Our dances connect us to our land, our dance connects us to our ancestors and our heritage. It could be also the conduit between ourselves and the spiritual realm. So what you're seeing, when you see haka is not just the physical representation, there's also a spiritual representation, a spiritual ceremony. That's also happening, taking place at that same time, through our voices, through the stamping on our ground, which represents the heartbeat of our earth mother, through the tiering of our clouds, through the raw emotion that you would have seen expressed in our faces and every single sinew in our body, every single molecule and part of our DNA connects to that moment. It's not just a dance.[126]

The spiritual connections that the haka enacts with the earth and other more-than-humans is again also apparent in the

Omaha Dance and the Jingle Dress Dance, which demonstrates the similarities among diverse Indigenous dances and understandings. As Te Ua expressed, these commonalities can cultivate solidarity among Indigenous peoples.[127]

The haka that Te Ua did provides a staunch critique of U.S. settler colonialism and DAPL from a Māori lens and through spiritual, ancestral expression. Unlike *Sioux Ghost Dance* and the Jingle Dress Dance Ceremony, Te Ua's haka was not planned, which is perhaps why the video that depicts him doing the haka is mostly shot from behind and in profile as opposed to directly from the front, which may have shown more expressiveness given the dance form. However, Te Ua's haka is still incredibly moving and powerful, which is why I have felt drawn to write about it since I first saw it circulating on social media in 2016. Te Ua also did not know he was being filmed or that the haka he did was posted online until after the fact.[128] Māori women with whom Te Ua was traveling had decided that they were going to go to a site where an action had happened a few days prior and offer their prayers and their respects to the land and the ancestors – according to Te Ua, to "show solidarity not just to the physical realm, but the spiritual realm as well."[129] However, Te Ua and the women had also been warned that "there was a sniper in the hills…and that they had live rounds [and]…had been giving instructions to use live rounds on us."[130] Based on this information, Te Ua decided he would accompany the women to protect them and stand in front of them as they walked to the site where they were going to pray. Shortly before the women finished praying, they heard an armored vehicle repeatedly rev its engine. At this time, the women began to retreat.[131] The women are not visible in a video of Te Ua's haka that has over 19,500 views on YouTube and over 5.6 million views on the AJ+ Facebook page with 93,000 reactions and 7,300 comments as of August 10, 2021.[132] Interestingly, similar to how the title *Sioux Ghost Dance* (mis)represents the dance by implying that the title of the film is the type of dance being depicted, the video of Te Ua's haka is labeled "New Zealand man performs Haka for Standing Rock Protestors in North Dakota," which simultaneously obscures Te Ua's Māori identity while reinforcing the authority and legitimacy of the settler state. Acclaimed Māori dancer, choreographer, and founding member of Atamira Dance Company, Jack Gray, also dissuaded me from using the word "performs" to describe haka; he wrote to me, "in our culture, we don't think of it as a performance so to speak. In our culture, haka (dance) is a way of expressing."[133]

In the video, snow falls lightly as Te Ua, wearing a ski jacket, black pants, and white Jordan 5 sneakers, paces back and forth on a highway – a lone Indigenous man facing an armored vehicle. He was emotional as he described,

> In that moment, I felt a feeling come over me, and I was trying to deny it. No, no, no. Not here, not here. And I felt myself dropping to my knees. And by that stage, I knew exactly what was happening is that my ancestors were using me as a vehicle or a vessel to send their support. Unrehearsed and unpracticed. I didn't even think about it. I went straight onto a haka that was composed by one of my grandfathers, which talks about the Treaty of Waitangi. Our treaty. The treaty that was signed in 1840 as a partnership between the Crown and our people and of course that was never honored. Never, ever. And as a result of that, our people were still facing the results of colonization through the position of our lands, our culture being totally and utterly ripped away from us through language, through different, extra laws and whatnot. So, what was going through my mind? I don't know. I can't tell you. What did happen was I became a vessel for the intention of the words to greet him, to pay homage to the ancestors of Standing Rock.[134]

## CONCLUSION

By charting the through lines of Lakota dances and lands on and as the frontlines, this chapter elucidates how Indigenous "histories" persist in the present given not only ongoing colonization, but also Indigenous peoples' resistance, resilience, and innovations. Broadly conceptualizing the frontlines can help to illuminate the overlaps, connections, discontinuities, and exclusions that can occur when theorizing colonization and Indigenous resistance – for example, how cinematic and even Native studies discourses[135] frequently disregard that *Sioux Ghost Dance*, shot at the Black Maria studio in Brooklyn, cannot be separated from the frontlines of Lenape people and lands. Indigenous dance is not a luxury, but a deeply contested space that has long been leveraged by non-Native and Native peoples to support, critique, and thwart settler colonialism. Indigenous people have utilized the cutting-edge technologies of their time to perpetuate, recast, and circulate their dances, and along with these dances, their dreams, prayers, and stories for the purposes of solidarity, social change, and survival. The Indigenous logics of respectful and reciprocal human and more-than-human interdependencies, which underpin each of the dances that I examine, is also at the heart of the NoDAPL and other Indigenous-led environmental movements.

In each of these dances, imprisonment and other forms of settler state violence pose a very real and present threat. Indigenous dance, in some cases, can be an alternative to armed resistance. As Nick Estes writes in regard to the Ghost Dancing, "[Wovoka's] call for peace was pragmatic: under present conditions, armed Indigenous resistance was futile."[136] The irony, however, is that Indigenous peoples endure some form of settler state brutality whether they resist or not, whether that violence – in the case of DAPL – is done to their bodies with "pepper spray, Tasers, rubber bullets, sound cannons, and batons against water protectors" or to the water, which is vital to their bodies.[137] Yet, Estes also writes: "What continues to sustain Indigenous peoples through the horrors of settler colonialism are the recent memories of freedom, the visions enacting it, and the daring conspiracies to recapture it."[138] What also sustains Indigenous peoples is hope for the future, including the embodied future of the next generation. I close with Lorde's words:

> Poetry coins the language to express and charter this revolutionary awareness and demand.... However,

experience has taught us that the action in the now is also always necessary. Our children cannot dream unless they live, they cannot live unless they are nourished, and who else will feed them the real food without which their dreams will be no different from ours?[139]

# FURTHER READING LIST

Brave Bird, Mary, and Richard Erdoes. *Lakota Woman*. New York: Grove Press, 1990. Narrated from the perspective of Mary Brave Bird, a Sicangu Lakota woman, this memoir provides further insight into how Lakota and other Native peoples have navigated and/or thwarted the structures of U.S. settler colonialism, including patriarchy. In particular, the text details Brave Bird's participation in the American Indian Movement, including her involvement in the 1972 Trail of Broken Treaties and the 1973 Indian Occupation at Wounded Knee.

Browner, Tara. *Heartbeat of the People: Music and Dance of the Northern Pow-Wow*. Champaign: University of Illinois Press, 2002. In this influential book, Tara Browner (Choctaw), an ethnomusicologist and Jingle Dress Dancer, draws on her own experiences as well as interviews with other pow-wow practitioners to delineate the history and politics of the Northern pow-wow of the Northern Plains and Great Lakes. The text contextualizes in detail a variety of tribally-specific and pan-Native American practices, including the Jingle Dress Dance, Omaha Dance, songs, and regalia, to demonstrate the capacities of pow-wow to produce tribal affiliation.

Hokowhitu, Brendan. "Haka: Colonized Physicality, Body-Logic, and Embodied Sovereignty." In *Performing Indigeneity: Global Histories and Contemporary Experiences*. Edited by H. Glenn Penny and Laura R. Graham, 273–304. Lincoln: University of Nebraska Press, 2014. This article by a Māori scholar discusses how colonizers in New Zealand have appropriated, leveraged, and (mis)represented haka for settler colonial and capitalist purposes while Māori peoples have danced the haka to enact self-representation/sovereignty. Given that discourses have frequently relegated Indigenous peoples and practices to the past, the author posits that doing the haka is a way of enacting sovereignty in the "immediate" present and forwarding Māori epistemologies specifically on the level of the body, which challenges Cartesian dualism.

Raheja, Michelle. "Visual Sovereignty." In *Native Studies Keywords*. Edited by Andrea Smith, Michelle Raheja, and Stephanie Nohelani Teves, 25–34. Tucson: University of Arizona Press, 2015. In this article, Michelle Raheja discusses the complex meanings of sovereignty – a central concept in Indigenous studies – in Native American/First Nations/Indigenous contexts. Although until recently, scholars have primarily written about sovereignty in the legal realm and social sciences and in ways that are recognizable to the settler state, the author emphasizes that broader and Native-centered understandings of sovereignty which often value creative and embodied forms of knowledge – such as Indigenous dance – are critical.

Shea Murphy, Jacqueline. *The People Have Never Stopped Dancing: Native American Modern Dance Histories*. Minneapolis: University of Minnesota Press, 2007. This innovative and comprehensive text presents the first book-length study of the history and politics of contemporary Native American dance. Some of what the author illuminates includes: how Native peoples have navigated U.S. prohibitions surrounding Indigenous movement modes; how "pioneering," non-Native, modern dance choreographers have appropriated Native dance forms and drawn on and profited from their (mis)conceptions about "Indianness"; the emergence of Aboriginal and Native American stage dance in the 1960s and 1970s; and the unique works of Indigenous choreographers today, which may also include commonalities among them, such as thematic concerns with the connections between past and present as well as human and more-than-human kin.

## TIMELINE

1876 – Battle of Greasy Grass occurs, when Lakota people, along with the Northern Cheyenne and Arapaho, defeat the 7th Cavalry Regiment.

1890 – Wounded Knee Massacre.

1972 – "Trail of Broken Treaties" march happens to Washington, D.C. and the subsequent occupation of the Bureau of Indian Affairs.

1973 – Wounded Knee Occupation, also referred to as a "Ghost Dance," occurs.

1978 – American Indian Religious Freedom Act ends previously banned Native dance.

# BIBLIOGRAPHY

"10-29-2016: JINGLE DRESS DANCERS AT THE FRONT-LINES, (EDITING NEEDED)." *Standing Rock Water Protector Camp Archive*. Accessed April 30, 2021. https://standingrockclassaction.org/?page_id=2736.

AJ+. "Haka for Standing Rock." *Facebook*. Video. November 29, 2016. www.facebook.com/watch/?v=847230752085100.

Baldy, Cutcha Risling. *We Are Dancing for You: Native Feminisms and the Revitalization of Women's Coming-of-Age Ceremonies*. Seattle: University of Washington Press, 2018.

Black Bear, Ben Jr. Interview with author. December 11, 2017.

Black Bear, Ben Sr. and R.D. Theisz. *Songs and Dances of the Lakota*. 2nd ed. Aberdeen: North Plains Press, 1984.

Blu Wakpa, Tria. "Challenging Settler Colonial Choreographies During COVID-19: Acosia Red

Elk's Powwow Yoga." *Critical Stages: The IATC Journal*, no. 23 (July 2021).

Blue Bird, George. Phone conversation with author. May 31, 2020.

Bold, Christine. "Early Cinematic Westerns." In *A History of Western American Literature*. Edited by Susan Kollin. Cambridge: Cambridge University Press, 2015.

Bolz, Peter. "The Lakota Sun Dance Between 1883 and 1997." In *Mirror Writing: (re-) constructions of Native American Identity*. Edited by Maria Moss and Thomas Claviez. Berlin and Cambridge: Galda +Wilch Verlag, 2000.

Branigin, Anne. "U.S. Poet Laureate Joy Harjo reflects on the lessons, rituals and gifts of the pandemic year." *The Lily*. April 17, 2020. www.thelily.com/us-poet-laureate-joy-harjo-reflects-on-the-lessons-rituals-and-gifts-of-the-pandemic-year/.

Brave Bird, Mary, and Richard Erdoes. *Lakota Woman*. New York, Grove Press, 1990.

Brown, Alleen, Will Parrish, and Alice Speri. "The Battle of Treaty Camp: Law Enforcement Descended on Standing Rock a Year Ago and Changed the DAPL Fight Forever." *The Intercept*. October 27, 2017. https://theintercept.com/2017/10/27/law-enforcement-descended-on-standing-rock-a-year-ago-and-changed-the-dapl-fight-forever/.

Brown, Toyacoyah. "Jingle Dress Dancers Bring Their Healing Dance to Standing Rock." *PowWows.com*. October 31, 2016. www.powwows.com/jingle-dress-dancers-bring-healing-dance-standing-rock/.

Browner, Tara. *Heartbeat of the People: Music and Dance of the Northern Pow-Wow*. Champaign: University of Illinois Press, 2002.

Creef, Elena Tajima, and Carl J. Petersen. "Remembering the Battle of Pezi Sla (Greasy Grass—aka Little Bighorn) with the Lakota, Northern Cheyenne, and Arapaho Victory Riders: An

Autoethnographic Photo Essay." *Cultural Studies ↔ Critical Methodologies* (2021): 1–14. DOI: 1532708621991128.

Crockford, Susannah. "Ghost Dance and Standing Rock Sioux." In *Critical Dictionary of Apocalyptic and Millenarian Movements.* Edited by James Crossley and Alastair Lockhart. January 15, 2021. Retrieved from www.cdamm.org/articles/standing-rock-sioux.

"Dancing for the Kinetograph: Buffalo Bill's Hyphenated Braves Immortalize Themselves." *The Sun.* September 25, 1894.

Darby, Jaye T., Courtney Elkin Mohler, and Christy Stanlake. *Critical Companion to Native American and First Nations Theatre and Performance.* Bloomsbury. 2020. Retrieved from www. bloomsbury.com/us/critical-companion-to-native-american-and-first-nations-theatre-and-performance-9781350035072/.

Davies, James Giago. "Native Sun News Today: A long history of stealing Lakota land." *Indianz.com.* April 8, 2019. www.indianz. com/News/2019/04/08/native-sun-news-today-a-long-history-of.asp.

Durham, Jimmie, and Jean Fisher. *A Certain Lack of Coherence: Writings on Art and Cultural Politics.* Kala Press, 1993.

Endres, Danielle. "American Indian Activism and Audience: Rhetorical Analysis of Leonard Peltier's Response to Denial of Clemency." *Communication Reports* 24, no. 1 (2011): 1–11.

Equal Justice Initiative. "Native American Activism." *Eji.org.* June 1, 2015.https://eji.org/news/history-racial-injustice-native-american-activism/.

Estes, Nick. *Our History is the Future: Standing Rock Versus the Dakota Access Pipeline, and the Long Tradition of Indigenous Resistance.* London: Verso, 2019.

Foster, Susan Leigh. *Choreographing Empathy: Kinesthesia in Performance.* New York: Routledge, 2011.

———. *Choreographing History.* Bloomington: Indiana University Press, 1995.

Gaudio, Michael. *Sound, Image, Silence: Art and the Aural Imagination in the Atlantic World.* Minneapolis: University of Minnesota Press, 2019.

Global News. "New Zealand man performs Haka for Standing Rock Protestors in North Dakota." *YouTube.* Video. November 29, 2016. www.youtube.com/watch?v=swv6hhsgxP0.

Gray, Jack. Correspondence with author. January 9, 2021.

Griffiths, Alison C. "Science and Spectacle: Native American Representation in Early Cinema." In *Dressing in Feathers: The Construction of American Popular Culture.* Boulder: Westview Press, 1996.

Gump, James O. "A Spirit of Resistance: Sioux, Xhosa, and Māori Responses to Western Dominance, 1840–1920." *Pacific Historical Review* 66, no. 1 (1997): 21–52.

Hall, Tonia Jo. "#NODAPL." *Facebook.* Video. October 29, 2016. www.facebook.com/100044388520755/videos/18688990-60004570.

Heise, William, Camera, Inc, Thomas A. Edison, and Hendricks. *Sioux Ghost Dance*. Produced by Dickson, W.K.-L., Uction (United States: Edison Manufacturing Co, 1894) Video. www.loc.gov/item/00694139/.

Hokowhitu, Brendan. "Haka: Colonized Physicality, Body-Logic, and Embodied Sovereignty." In *Performing Indigeneity: Global Histories and Contemporary Experiences*. Edited by H. Glenn Penny and Laura R. Graham, 273–304. Lincoln: University of Nebraska Press, 2014.

Huhndorf, Shari M. *Going Native: Indians in the American Cultural Imagination*. Ithaca and London: Cornell University Press, 2001.

___. *Mapping the Americas: The Transnational Politics of Contemporary Native Culture*. Ithaca and London: Cornell University Press, 2009.

IMDb. "Dances with Wolves: Filming & Production." *IMDb. com*. Accessed April 30, 2021. www.imdb.com/title/tt0099348/locations.

Jackson, Steven J., and Brendan Hokowhitu. "Sport, Tribes, and Technology: The New Zealand All Blacks Haka and the Politics of Identity." *Journal of Sport and Social Issues* 26, no. 2 (2002): 125–139.

Johnson, Troy. "We Hold The Rock: The Alcatraz Indian Occupation." *National Park Service* online. November 26, 2019. www.nps.gov/alca/learn/historyculture/we-hold-the-rock.htm.

Killsback, Leo. "Crowns of Honor: Sacred Laws of Eagle-Feather War Bonnets and Repatriating the Icon of the Great Plains." *Great Plains Quarterly* 33, no. 1 (2013): 1–23.

Library of Congress. "Sioux Ghost Dance." *LOC.gov*. www.loc.gov/item/00694139/.

Liu, Marian. "A culture, not a costume: How to handle cultural appropriation during Halloween." *The Washington Post*. October 30, 2019. www.washingtonpost.com/nation/2019/10/30/culture-not-costume/.

Lorde, Audre. *Sister Outsider: Essays and Speeches*. Berkeley: Crossing Press, 2007.

___. *The Selected Works of Audre Lorde*. Edited by Roxane Gay. W.W. Norton & Company, 2020.

Matson, William B. *Crazy Horse: The Lakota Warrior's Life & Legacy*. Gibbs Smith, 2016.

McCully, Betsy. *City at the Water's Edge: A Natural History of New York*. New Brunswick: Rutgers University Press, 2020.

Moore, Laura Jane. "Elle Meets the President: Weaving Navajo Culture and Commerce in the Southwestern Tourist Industry." *Frontiers: A Journal of Women Studies* 22, No. 1 (2001): 21–44. DOI: www.jstor.org/stable/3347066.

Moses, Lester George. *Wild West Shows and the Images of American Indians, 1883–1933*. Albuquerque: University of New Mexico Press, 1999.

Moya-Smith, Simon (@SimonMoyaSmith). "Jingle Dress dancers took to the front line at Standing Rock in North Dakota Saturday…" *Twitter*. Video. October 29, 2016. https://twitter.com/simonmoyasmith/status/792483544639561728?lang=en.

Mutu, Margaret. "Māori issues." *The Contemporary Pacific* 27, no. 1 (2015): 273–281.

O'Brien, Jean M. *Firsting and Lasting: Writing Indians Out of Existence in New England*. Minneapolis: University of Minnesota Press, 2010.

Peters, Evelyn, and Chris Andersen, eds. *Indigenous in the City: Contemporary Identities and Cultural Innovation*. Vancouver: UBC Press, 2013.

Prins, Harald E.L. "Visual Anthropology." In *A Companion to the Anthropology of American Indians*. Edited by Thomas Biolsi, 506–525. Malden, MA: Blackwell Publishing, 2004.

Raheja, Michelle H. *Reservation Reelism: Redfacing, Visual Sovereignty, and Representations of Native Americans in Film*. Lincoln: University of Nebraska Press, 2013.

____. "Visual Sovereignty." In *Native Studies Keywords*. Edited by Andrea Smith, Michelle Raheja, and Stephanie Nohelani Teves, 25–34. Tucson: University of Arizona Press, 2015.

Red Elk, Acosia. Interview with author. June 18, 2020.

"Red Men Again Conquered." *New York Herald*. September 25, 1894.

Rivas, Josué. "Black Liberation and Indigenous Sovereignty Are Interconnected." *The Nation*. June 29, 2021. www.thenation.com/article/politics/black-liberation-indigenous-sovereignty/.

Roberts, Kathleen Glenister. "War, Masculinity, and Native Americans." In *Global Masculinities and Manhood*. Edited by Ronald J. Jackson and Murali Balaji, 141–160. Champaign, IL: University of Illinois Press, 2013.

Rony, Fatimah Tobing. *The Third Eye: Race, Cinema, and Ethnographic Spectacle*. Durham: Duke University Press, 1996.

Schechner, Richard. *Between Theater and Anthropology*. Philadelphia: University of Pennsylvania Press, 1985.

Shea Murphy, Jacqueline. *The People Have Never Stopped Dancing: Native American Modern Dance Histories*. Minneapolis: University of Minnesota Press, 2007.

Simmon, Scott. *The Invention of Western Film: A Cultural History of the Genre's First Half Century*. Cambridge: Cambridge University Press, 2003.

Speed, Shannon. *Incarcerated Stories: Indigenous Women Migrants and Violence in the Settler-Capitalist State*. Chapel Hill: University of North Carolina Press, 2019.

Spehr, Paul. *The Man Who Made Movies: W.K.L. Dickson*. New Barnet: John Libbey Publishing Ltd, 2008.

Tahmahkera, Dustin. *Tribal Television: Viewing Native People in Sitcoms*. Chapel Hill: University of North Carolina Press, 2014.

Tapahe, Erin. "This morning at Standing Rock, many women participated in a sacred ceremonial Women's Jingle dance and this was the first time it was allowed to be recorded…" *Facebook*. Video. October 29, 2016. www.facebook.com/erin.tapahe/videos/1220201151355408/.

Te Ua, Kereama. Interview with author, March 9, 2021.

"The Longest Walk," *American Indian Journal* 4, no. 9 (September 1978): 17–30.

The William F. Cody Archive. "No Neck, Johnny Burke, 1883–1921." Accessed April 30, 2021. https://codyarchive.org/life/wfc.person.html#noneck.j.

Thiel, Mark G. "Origins of the Jingle Dress Dance." *Whispering Wind* 36, no. 5 (2007): 14–18.

___. "The Omaha Dance in Oglala and Sicangu Sioux History." *Whispering Wind* 23, no. 5 (Fall/Winter 1990): 4–17.

Todd, Zoe. "Refracting the state through human-fish relations." *Decolonization: Indigeneity, Education & Society* 7, no. 1 (2018): 60–75.

Tuck, Eve, and K. Wayne Yang. "Decolonization is not a metaphor." *Decolonization: Indigeneity, Education & Society* 1, no. 1 (2012): 1–40.

Verhoeff, Nanna. "MOVING INDIANS: Deconstructing the Other in Moving Images." *Native American Studies*, 2007.

"War Dances Before It: Buffalo Bill's Indians Exhibit for the Wonderful Kinetoscope Future Generations to See Weird Sight Presented by the Red Men of the Far West." *New York Press*. September 25, 1894.

Warren, Louis S. *Buffalo Bill's America: William Cody and The Wild West Show*. New York: Vintage Books, 2005.

# NOTES

1 Susan Leigh Foster, *Choreographing History* (Bloomington: Indiana University Press, 1995), 3.

2 Eve Tuck and K. Wayne Yang, "Decolonization is not a metaphor," *Decolonization: Indigeneity, Education & Society* 1, no. 1 (2012): 4–5.

3 Audre Lorde, *The Selected Works of Audre Lorde*, ed. Roxane Gay (New York: W.W. Norton & Company, 2020).

4 Audre Lorde, *Sister Outsider: Essays and Speeches* (Berkeley: Crossing Press, 2007), 37.

5 Eve Tuck and K. Wayne Yang, "Decolonization is not a metaphor," 5; Zoe Todd, "Refracting the state through

human-fish relations," *Decolonization: Indigeneity, Education & Society* 7, no. 1 (2018): 66.

6 Shannon Speed, *Incarcerated Stories: Indigenous Women Migrants and Violence in the Settler-Capitalist State* (Chapel Hill: University of North Carolina Press, 2019), 15.

7 Jacqueline Shea Murphy, *The People Have Never Stopped Dancing: Native American Modern Dance Histories* (University of Minnesota Press, 2007), 199.

8 Cutcha Risling Baldy, *We Are Dancing for You: Native Feminisms and the Revitalization of Women's Coming-of-Age Ceremonies* (Seattle: University of Washington Press, 2018), 9.

9 Susan Leigh Foster, *Choreographing Empathy: Kinesthesia in Performance* (New York: Routledge, 2011), 10.

10 Eve Tuck and K. Wayne Yang, "Decolonization is not a metaphor," 5.

11 Evelyn Peters and Chris Andersen, eds., *Indigenous in the City: Contemporary Identities and Cultural Innovation* (Vancouver: UBC Press, 2013), 2.

12 Anne Branigin, "U.S. Poet Laureate Joy Harjo reflects on the lessons, rituals and gifts of the pandemic year," *The Lily*, April 17, 2020, www.thelily.com/us-poet-laureate-joy-harjo-reflects-on-the-lessons-rituals-and-gifts-of-the-pandemic-year/.

13 Josué Rivas, "Black Liberation and Indigenous Sovereignty Are Interconnected," *The Nation*, June 29, 2021, www.thenation.com/article/politics/black-liberation-indigenous-sovereignty/.

14 Tria Blu Wakpa, "Challenging Settler Colonial Choreographies During COVID-19: Acosia Red Elk's Powwow Yoga," *Critical Stages: The IATC Journal*, no. 23 (July 2021).

15 Jacqueline Shea Murphy, *The People Have Never Stopped Dancing*, 29–31.

16 Richard Schechner, "Restoration of Behavior," in *Between Theater and Anthropology* (Philadelphia: University of Pennsylvania Press, 1985).

17 Eve Tuck and K. Wayne Yang, "Decolonization is not a metaphor," 12.

18 Susannah Crockford, "Ghost Dance and Standing Rock Sioux," In *Critical Dictionary of Apocalyptic and Millenarian Movements*, edited by James Crossley and Alastair Lockhart, January 15, 2021. Retrieved from www.cdamm.org/articles/standing-rock-sioux, 2.

19 Jacqueline Shea Murphy, *The People Have Never Stopped Dancing*, 72.

20 James O. Gump, "A Spirit of Resistance: Sioux, Xhosa, and Māori Responses to Western Dominance, 1840–1920," *Pacific Historical Review* 66, no. 1 (1997): 22.

21 Jean M. O'Brien, *Firsting and Lasting: Writing Indians Out of Existence in New England*, (Minneapolis: University of Minnesota Press, 2010), xiii.

22 Margaret Matu, "Māori issues," *The Contemporary Pacific* 27, no. 1 (2015): 274.

23 James Giago Davies, "Native Sun News Today: A long history of stealing Lakota land," *Indianz.com*, April 8, 2019, www.indianz.com/News/2019/04/08/native-sun-news-today-a-long-history-of.asp.

24 Elena Tajima Creef and Carl J. Petersen, "Remembering the Battle of Pezi Sla (Greasy Grass—aka Little Bighorn) with the Lakota, Northern Cheyenne, and Arapaho Victory Riders: An Autoethnographic Photo Essay," *Cultural Studies ↔ Critical Methodologies* (2021): 1, DOI: 1532708621991128.

25 Jacqueline Shea Murphy, *The People Have Never Stopped Dancing*, 29.

26 Jacqueline Shea Murphy, *The People Have Never Stopped Dancing*, 40; Peter Bolz, "The Lakota Sun Dance Between 1883 and 1997," In *Mirror Writing: (re-) constructions of Native American Identity*, edited by Maria Moss and Thomas Claviez (Berlin and Cambridge: Galda +Wilch Verlag, 2000), 1.

27 Jacqueline Shea Murphy, *The People Have Never Stopped Dancing*, 73–74.

28 Harald E.L. Prins, "Visual Anthropology," In *A Companion to the Anthropology of American Indians*, Edited by Thomas Biolsi (Malden, MA: Blackwell Publishing, 2004), 521.

29 Lester George Moses, *Wild West Shows and the Images of American Indians, 1883–1933* (Albuquerque: University of New Mexico Press, 1999), 4–5.

30 Shannon Speed, *Incarcerated Stories*, 15.

31 Louis S. Warren, *Buffalo Bill's America: William Cody and The Wild West Show* (New York: Vintage Books, 2005), 364–265; Jaye T. Darby, Courtney Elkin Mohler, and Christy Stanlake, *Critical Companion to Native American and First Nations Theatre and Performance.* (Bloomsbury: 2020), retrieved from www.bloomsbury.com/us/critical-companion-to-native-american-and-first-nations-theatre-and-performance-9781350035072/, 29–30.

32 Jacqueline Shea Murphy, *The People Have Never Stopped Dancing*, 75.

33 Jacqueline Shea Murphy, *The People Have Never Stopped Dancing*, 75.

34 Troy Johnson, "We Hold The Rock: The Alcatraz Indian Occupation," *National Park Service* online, November 26, 2019, www.nps.gov/alca/learn/historyculture/we-hold-the-rock.htm; Mary Brave Bird and Richard Erdoes, *Lakota Woman* (New York, Grove Press, 1990), 133–135; Equal Justice Initiative, "Native American Activism," *Eji.org*, June 1, 2015, https://eji.org/news/history-racial-injustice-native-american-activism/.

35 Susannah Crockford, "Ghost Dance and Standing Rock Sioux," 2.

36 "The Longest Walk," *American Indian Journal* 4, no. 9 (September 1978): 18.

37 Danielle Endres, "American Indian Activism and Audience: Rhetorical Analysis of Leonard Peltier's Response to Denial of Clemency," *Communication Reports* 24, no. 1 (2011): 10.

38 Mary Brave Bird and Richard Erdoes, *Lakota Woman*, 133–135.

39 Dustin Tahmahkera, *Tribal Television: Viewing Native People in Sitcoms* (Chapel Hill: University of North Carolina Press, 2014), 102; IMDb, "Dances with Wolves: Filming & Production," *IMDb.com*, accessed April 30, 2021, www.imdb.com/title/tt0099348/locations.

40 Shari M. Huhndorf, *Going Native: Indians in the American Cultural Imagination* (Ithaca and London: Cornell University Press, 2001), 3.

41 Susannah Crockford, "Ghost Dance and Standing Rock Sioux," 1.

42 Susannah Crockford, "Ghost Dance and Standing Rock Sioux," 2.

43 William Heise, Camera, Inc, Thomas A. Edison, and Hendricks, *Sioux Ghost Dance*, Produced by Dickson, W.K.-L., Uction (United States: Edison Manufacturing Co, 1894) Video, www.loc.gov/item/00694139/.

44 William Heise, Camera, Inc, Thomas A. Edison, and Hendricks, *Sioux Ghost Dance*.

45 "Dancing for the Kinetograph: Buffalo Bill's Hyphenated Braves Immortalize Themselves," *The Sun*, September 25, 1894; "War Dances Before It: Buffalo Bill's Indians Exhibit for the Wonderful Kinetoscope Future Generations to See Weird Sight Presented by the Red Men of the Far West," *New York Press*, September 25, 1894.

46 "Red Men Again Conquered," *New York Herald*, September 25, 1894.

47 Michael Gaudio, *Sound, Image, Silence: Art and the Aural Imagination in the Atlantic World* (Minneapolis: University of Minnesota Press, 2019), 145.

48 Michael Gaudio, *Sound, Image, Silence: Art and the Aural Imagination in the Atlantic World*, 126.

49 Michael Gaudio, *Sound, Image, Silence: Art and the Aural Imagination in the Atlantic World*, 125.

50 William B. Matson, *Crazy Horse: The Lakota Warrior's Life & Legacy* (Gibbs Smith, 2016) 94–96, 421.

51 Harald E.L. Prins, "Visual Anthropology," 521.

52 Michael Gaudio, *Sound, Image, Silence: Art and the Aural Imagination in the Atlantic World*, xviii; Christine Bold, "Early Cinematic Westerns," in *A History of Western American Literature*, edited by Susan Kollin (Cambridge: Cambridge University Press, 2015), 225–226.

53 Jacqueline Shea Murphy, *The People Have Never Stopped Dancing*, 29; Michael Gaudio, *Sound, Image, Silence: Art and the Aural Imagination in the Atlantic World*, 127.

54  Fatimah Tobing Rony, *The Third Eye: Race, Cinema, and Ethnographic Spectacle* (Durham: Duke University Press, 1996), 91–93.

55  Shari M. Huhndorf, *Going Native: Indians in the American Cultural Imagination*, 27–28.

56  Mark G. Thiel, "The Omaha Dance in Oglala and Sicangu Sioux History," *Whispering Wind* 23, no. 5 (1990): 5.

57  Nick Estes, *Our History is the Future*, 68–69.

58  "War Dances Before It"; "Red Men Again Conquered."

59  Black Bear, Ben Jr., Interview with author; Ben Black Bear, Sr. and R.D. Theisz, *Songs and Dances of the Lakota* 2nd ed. (Aberdeen: North Plains Press, 1894), 19, 37.

60  Ben Black Bear, Sr. and R.D. Theisz, *Songs and Dances of the Lakota*, 19, 37.

61  Michael Gaudio, *Sound, Image, Silence: Art and the Aural Imagination in the Atlantic World*, 131.

62  Michael Gaudio, *Sound, Image, Silence: Art and the Aural Imagination in the Atlantic World*, 131.

63  Library of Congress, "Sioux Ghost Dance," *LOC.gov*, www.loc.gov/item/00694139/.

64  Library of Congress. "Sioux Ghost Dance"; Jacqueline Shea Murphy, *The People Have Never Stopped Dancing*, 75.

65  Michael Gaudio, *Sound, Image, Silence: Art and the Aural Imagination in the Atlantic World*, 133.

66  Michael Gaudio, *Sound, Image, Silence: Art and the Aural Imagination in the Atlantic World*, 126.

67  Library of Congress, "Sioux Ghost Dance"; Marian Liu, "A culture, not a costume: How to handle cultural appropriation during Halloween," *The Washington Post*, October 30, 2019, www.washingtonpost.com/nation/2019/10/30/culture-not-costume/.

68  Mark G. Thiel, "The Omaha Dance in Oglala and Sicangu Sioux History," 5.

69  Michael Gaudio, *Sound, Image, Silence: Art and the Aural Imagination in the Atlantic World*, 180.

70  Michelle H. Raheja, *Reservation Reelism: Redfacing, Visual Sovereignty, and Representations of Native Americans in Film* (Lincoln: University of Nebraska Press, 2013).

71  The William F. Cody Archive, "No Neck, Johnny Burke, 1883–1921," Accessed April 30, 2021, https://codyarchive.org/life/wfc.person.html#noneck.j; A four-month-old baby girl, Zintkala Nuni, also lived (81–82); Betsy McCully, *City at the Water's Edge: A Natural History of New York* (New Brunswick: Rutgers University Press, 2020).

72  "War Dances Before It"; William Heise, Camera, Inc, Thomas A. Edison, and Hendricks, *Sioux Ghost Dance.*

73  Laura Jane Moore, "Elle Meets the President: Weaving Navajo Culture and Commerce in the Southwestern Tourist Industry," *Frontiers: A Journal of Women Studies* 22, No. 1 (2001): 30, DOI: www.jstor.org/stable/3347066.

74 Blue Bird, George. Phone conversation with author. May 31, 2020 ; Leo Killsback, "Crowns of Honor: Sacred Laws of Eagle-Feather War Bonnets and Repatriating the Icon of the Great Plains," *Great Plains Quarterly* 33, no. 1 (2013): 8.

75 Shari M. Huhndorf, *Going Native: Indians in the American Cultural Imagination.*

76 Brendan Hokowhitu, "Haka: Colonized Physicality, Body-Logic, and Embodied Sovereignty," In *Performing Indigeneity: Global Histories and Contemporary Experiences,* edited by H. Glenn Penny and Laura R. Graham, 295–296; Michelle Raheja, "Visual Sovereignty," In *Native Studies Keywords,* edited by Andrea Smith, Michelle Raheja, and Stephanie Nohelani Teves (Tucson: University of Arizona Press, 2015), 27–28.

77 Michael Gaudio, *Sound, Image, Silence: Art and the Aural Imagination in the Atlantic World,* 128.

78 Leo Killsback, "Crowns of Honor," 8.

79 Leo Killsback, "Crowns of Honor," 16.

80 Leo Killsback, "Crowns of Honor," 3, 8–9.

81 Leo Killsback, "Crowns of Honor," 3.

82 Leo Killsback, "Crowns of Honor," 19-20.

83 Kathleen Glenister Roberts, "War, Masculinity, and Native Americans," In *Global Masculinities and Manhood,* edited by Ronald J. Jackson and Murali Balaji (Champaign, IL: University of Illinois Press, 2013), 142.

84 Jimmie Durham and Jean Fisher, *A Certain Lack of Coherence: Writings on Art and Cultural Politics* (Kala Press, 1993), 11.

85 William Heise, Camera, Inc, Thomas A. Edison, and Hendricks, *Sioux Ghost Dance*; Library of Congress, "Sioux Ghost Dance," *LOC.gov,* www.loc.gov/item/00694139/.

86 Michael Gaudio, *Sound, Image, Silence: Art and the Aural Imagination in the Atlantic World,* 126; Mark G. Thiel, "The Omaha Dance in Oglala and Sicangu Sioux History."

87 "War Dances Before It."

88 Alleen Brown, Will Parrish, and Alice Speri, "The Battle of Treaty Camp: Law Enforcement Descended on Standing Rock a Year Ago and Changed the DAPL Fight Forever," *The Intercept,* October 27, 2017; Nick Estes, *Our History is the Future: Standing Rock Versus the Dakota Access Pipeline, and the Long Tradition of Indigenous Resistance* (London: Verso, 2019), 2.

89 Alleen Brown, Will Parrish, and Alice Speri, "The Battle of Treaty Camp."

90 Nick Estes, *Our History is the Future,* 43, 37.

91 Alleen Brown, Will Parrish, and Alice Speri, "The Battle of Treaty Camp."

92 Toyacoyah Brown, "Jingle Dress Dancers Bring Their Healing Dance to Standing Rock," *PowWows.com,* October 31, 2016, www.powwows.com/jingle-dress-dancers-bring-healing-dance-standing-rock/.

93  Mark G. Thiel, "Origins of the Jingle Dress Dance," 14.

94  Audre Lorde, *Sister Outsider*, 37.

95  Mark G. Thiel, "Origins of the Jingle Dress Dance," 16.

96  Mark G. Thiel, "Origins of the Jingle Dress Dance," 16.

97  Mark G. Thiel, "Origins of the Jingle Dress Dance," 16.

98  Nick Estes, *Our History is the Future*, 14.

99  Tara Browner, *Heartbeat of the People: Music and Dance of the Northern Pow-Wow* (Champaign: University of Illinois Press, 2002), 55.

100 Acosia Red Elk, Interview with author, June 18, 2020.

101 Acosia Red Elk, Interview with author.

102 Acosia Red Elk, Interview with author.

103 Acosia Red Elk, Interview with author.

104 Alleen Brown, Will Parrish, and Alice Speri, "The Battle of Treaty Camp."

105 "10-29-2016: JINGLE DRESS DANCERS AT THE FRONTLINES, (EDITING NEEDED)," *Standing Rock Water Protector Camp Archive*, accessed April 30, 2021, https:// standingrockclassaction.org/?page_id=2736; Erin Tapahe, "This morning at Standing Rock, many women participated in a sacred ceremonial Women's Jingle dance and this was the first time it was allowed to be recorded..." *Facebook*, Video, October 29, 2016, www.facebook.com/erin.tapahe/videos/ 1220201151355408/.

106 Erin Tapahe, "This morning at Standing Rock."

107 Erin Tapahe, "This morning at Standing Rock."

108 Simon Moya-Smith (@SimonMoyaSmith), "Jingle Dress dancers took to the front line at Standing Rock in North Dakota Saturday..." *Twitter*, Video, October 29, 2016.

109 Tonia Jo Hall, "#NODAPL," *Facebook*, Video, October 29, 2016, www.facebook.com/100044388520755/videos/ 1868899060004570.

110 Tonia Jo Hall, "#NODAPL."

111 Tonia Jo Hall, "#NODAPL."

112 James O. Gump, "A Spirit of Resistance," 22, 47.

113 James O. Gump, "A Spirit of Resistance," 24.

114 James O. Gump, "A Spirit of Resistance," 30.

115 James O. Gump, "A Spirit of Resistance," 32.

116 James O. Gump, "A Spirit of Resistance," 33–34.

117 Kereama Te Ua, Interview with author, March 9, 2021.

118 James O. Gump, "A Spirit of Resistance," 35, 37.

119 Brendan Hokowhitu, "Haka: Colonized Physicality, Body-Logic, and Embodied Sovereignty," 279.

120 Brendan Hokowhitu, "Haka: Colonized Physicality, Body-Logic, and Embodied Sovereignty," 277.

121 Steven J. Jackson and Brendan Hokowhitu, "Sport, Tribes, and Technology: The New Zealand All Blacks Haka and the Politics of Identity," *Journal of Sport and Social Issues* 26, no. 2 (2002): 128; Mark G. Thiel, "Origins of the Jingle Dress

Dance"; "The Omaha Dance in Oglala and Sicangu Sioux History," *Whispering Wind* 23, no. 5 (Fall/Winter 1990): 5.

122  Brendan Hokowhitu, "Haka: Colonized Physicality, Body-Logic, and Embodied Sovereignty," 296–298.

123  Nick Estes, *Our History is the Future*, 15; Kereama Te Ua, Interview with author, March 9, 2021.

124  Kereama Te Ua, Interview with author, March 9, 2021.

125  Kereama Te Ua, Interview with author.

126  Kereama Te Ua, Interview with author.

127  Kereama Te Ua, Interview with author.

128  Kereama Te Ua, Interview with author.

129  Kereama Te Ua, Interview with author.

130  Kereama Te Ua, Interview with author.

131  Kereama Te Ua, Interview with author.

132  AJ+, "Haka for Standing Rock," *Facebook*, Video, November 29, 2016.

133  Jack Gray, Correspondence with author, January 9, 2021.

134  Kereama Te Ua, Interview with author, March 9, 2021.

135  Christine Bold, "Early Cinematic Westerns,"; Michael Gaudio, *Sound, Image, Silence: Art and the Aural Imagination in the Atlantic World*; Alison Griffiths, "Science and Spectacle: Native American Representation in Early Cinema," in *Dressing in Feathers: The Construction of the American Popular Culture* (Boulder: Westview, 1996); Scott Simmon, *The Invention of the Western Film: A Cultural History of the Genre's First Half Century* (Cambridge: Cambridge University Press, 2003); Paul Spehr, *The Man Who Made Movies: W.K.L. Dickson* (New Barnet: John Libbey Publishing Ltd, 2008); Nanna Verhoeff, "MOVING INDIANS: Deconstructing the *Other* in Moving Images," *Native American Studies* 21.1 (2007); Louis S. Warren, *Buffalo Bill's America*.

136  Nick Estes, *Our History is the Future*, 246.

137  Alleen Brown, Will Parrish, and Alice Speri, "The Battle of Treaty Camp."

138  Nick Estes, *Our History is the Future*, 258.

139  Audre Lorde, *Sister Outsider: Essays and Speeches*, 37.

# CHAPTER 2

# Silk Road

## Commerce, Conquest, and College

*Laurel Victoria Gray*

The romanticized term *Silk Road* conjures up images of camel caravans crossing vast expanses of desert, but this dynamic, trans-Eurasian trade conduit did more than connect Europe and China.[1]

It also enabled regional commerce between Asia's nomadic and settled communities. True, silk was a sought-after luxury item, but much more than silk and other prized goods traveled the network of trade routes. Ideas, languages, art, technology, and religions moved back and forth along these caravan trails, as well as people with their own spiritual practices, languages, customs, cuisine – and dance. Many of the civilizations where the dances originated are now gone, but these uprooted traditions crossed cultures to adapt and thrive in new lands where they inspired poets, enchanted emperors, and even empowered college students.

## THE SOGDIAN MERCHANTS

Commercial agents of cultural transmission, the Sogdians succeeded as Silk Road merchants. They came from the territory of modern-day Uzbekistan and Tajikistan, from the cities of Bukhara, Samarkand, and Penjikent. Sogdian trade with China peaked between 500 to 800 CE, catering to the T'ang Dynasty's taste for imported luxuries, such as gemstones, horses, grape wine, precious metals, amber, furs, slaves, and foreign dancers.[2] Speaking an Iranian language, these merchants created permanent enclaves in the

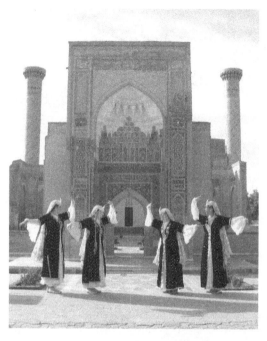

**Figure 2.1:** Silk Road Dance Company in Uzbek dance pose, Samarkand, Uzbekistan, in front of Gur Emir, tomb of Tamerlane, August 2005. Photographer: Laurel Victoria Gray.

prosperous city of Chang'an, the T'ang capital, which was then one of the largest cities in the world. Sogdians were considered by the Chinese as *hu*, "Western barbarians," and were the largest non-Chinese community at the time.[3] They also received Chinese names but, instead of being identified with a particular family or clan as was done in Chinese nomenclature, they were given surnames that reflected their place of origin, i.e., *An* for Bukhara, *Chach* for Tashkent, and *Kang* for Samarkand.[4] Identified by these place-names, Sogdians also stood out with their Western features – deep set eyes, thick beards, prominent noses, and unique clothing. Although they sometimes married Chinese women, they clung to other aspects of their culture, including language and religion, even building Zoroastrian fire temples for their émigré communities.

T'ang tastes for foreign imports included dancers; professional performers from the Sogdian Central Asian homeland were brought to Chang'an. According to an account in the T'ang Annals, Central Asian dancing girls were sent "from Samarkand as tribute to the Chinese Court."[5] The aristocracy found these performers captivating, labelling their dances as either "pliant" or "vigorous."[6] In one dramatic duet, two young girls from Chach (Tashkent) emerged from the opening petals of artificial lotuses to dance to driving drum rhythms. They wore hats decorated with golden bells and slippers made from red brocade. The celebrated Chinese poet, Bai Juyi, recorded his impression:

> I watch – too soon the tune is done, they will not be detained;
>
> Whirling in clouds, escorted by rain, they are off to the Terrace of the Sun.[7]

Another dance included mulberry branches, an interesting connection with silk manufacture since mulberry leaves are the primary food source of silkworms, essential to the development of their cocoons. Other dancers, in an acrobatic feat, performed on top of spinning balls.[8] Enslaved Persian women were sold into Chang'an "pleasure houses" where their dance performances comprised some of the entertainment available to clients.

A lively dance, the *huteng wu*, performed by "foreign barbarian" boys included leaping and turning, as well as a connection to wine.

> The Iranian from Tashkent appears young.
>
> He dances to the music holding the wine goblet, as rapid as a bird.
>
> He wears a cloth cap of foreign make, empty and pointed at the top,
>
> His Iranian robe of fine felt has tight sleeves.
>
> Liu Yanshi (d. 812)[9]

A "whirling" dance which they brought from their homeland created such a sensation in Chang'an that it could rightfully be called a dance craze. T'ang art depicts Sogdians feasting and drinking, with men performing this dance, spinning in place, often on a small circular carpet. An image of a whirling dancer appears on the funerary couch of the Sogdian man identified as An Qie, a *sabao* or caravan leader.[10] His Chinese-assigned surname "An" connects him to the Central Asian city of Bukhara where a present-day dance tradition also includes impressive spins.

Women also performed the Sogdian whirl. Buddhist art from this era portrays female *apsaras*, or spirits of the clouds and water, turning in a similar manner, with silk streamers creating a delayed line in the air as they rotated. The poet Bai Juyi described it.

> *Iranian whirling girl, Iranian whirling girl…*
>
> *At the sound of the string and drums, she raises her arms,*
>
> *Like swirling snowflakes tossed about, she turns in her twirling dance.*
>
> *Whirling to the left, turning to the right, she never feels exhausted,*
>
> *A thousand rounds, ten thousand circuits—it never seems to end…*
>
> *Compared to her, the wheels of a racing chariot revolve slowly and a whirlwind is sluggish.*
>
> *Iranian whirling girl,*
>
> *You came from Sogdiana…*[11]

This "Sogdian whirl" became such a fad that even some Chinese court officials performed it, which apparently raised eyebrows of those who thought it undignified for **courtiers** to take up a foreign dance.[12] Bai Juyi's poem describes the dance as so popular that "officials and concubines all learned how to circle and turn."[13] Reputedly, the T'ang Emperor Xuanzong (ruled 712–756 CE) was so enraptured by a performance of the whirling dance by Yang Guifei, one of his 3,000 concubines, that he made her his favorite. In Bai Juyi's famous narrative poem, *Song of Everlasting Sorrow*, a roman-ticized retelling of the love-affair between Xuanzong and Lady Yang, describes the emperor as so captivated by this concubine that he abandoned all affairs of state, endangering the empire.[14]

Size seems to have placed no barrier on performers. General An Lushan excelled at the Sogdian whirling dance even though he reportedly weighed 400 pounds. He was known to be non-Chinese of Turco-Sogdian ancestry; his name "An" suggests a connection with Bukhara.[15] This dancing general launched a bloody rebellion in 755 CE to overthrow the Chinese emperor that slaughtered armies and impacted the civilian population through famine and displacement. By the time the rebellion was finally subdued in 763 CE, with the help of Arab and Uyghur forces, all three – Yang Guifei, Emperor Xuanzong, and An Lushan – were dead, as well as many as 36 million people.[16]

What happened to the Sogdians and their whirling dance? After the rebellion of the General An Lushan, the ancient tension between Chinese and *hu* became more manifest. The open and cosmopolitan nature of Chang'an changed; foreigners and foreign ideas began to be regarded with suspi-cion. Sogdians began to hide their origins and to assimilate. Furthermore, to the west, the Muslim Arab conquest of the Persian Sasanian Empire in 651 CE impacted Sogdian homelands and endangered **Zoroastrianism**.

But Sogdians did not disappear completely. The Yaghnobi people, who currently live in a remote area of Tajikistan, speak a dialect which connects them to the ancient Sogdians. As for the Sogdian dances, alluring traces exist in the modern day. In Tajikistan's Pamir mountains, a distinctive and mesmerizing dance called *Rapo* incorporates a series of spins which continually change rotational direction, just as described in Bai Juyi's poem.

In Bukhara, once a center for Sogdian population – and likely hereditary home of General An Lushan – an interest-ing spinning tradition still exists. One kind of turn, called *shokh*, is a quick 360-degree turn done in place, achieved by pushing off with one foot while pivoting on the other, similar to images of Sogdian dancers found in T'ang art. Another turn is called *charkh*, which is the Persian word for "wheel." In executing *charkh*, the dancer sometimes leans forward with the upper torso while turning, creating a **sagittal** path.

And among Persian and Azeri men, a furiously fast spin – also called *charkh* – is done as part of the athletic training that takes place in the *Zurkhaneh* gymnasium, or "Houses of Strength." Accompanied by drumming on the *zarb* and the chanting of epic poetry, vigorous workouts in the *zurkhaneh* connect to pre-Islamic spiritual traditions.

Another turning practice, deeply connected to the Persian poet and theologian Jalaleddin Rumi, continues today with the Mevlevi Sufis of Konya, Turkey, known as "whirling dervishes." The spiritual ceremony called *sema* is a ritual with several sections, the most dramatic of which is "the turn," in which the individual participants, or *semazens*, turn continuously in place, always to the left "over the heart." And here, again, the Persian term *charkh* - written as *çark* in Turkish – is used to describe the characteristic rotation. The typically white clothing of the *semazen* consists of a huge, long skirt (*tenure*) with a weighted hem that gradually opens wide when spinning begins. This tradition also exists in Egypt where it is called *tanoura*, a term which denotes the dance, the dancer, and the characteristic skirt of the costume.[17]

The Sogdian legacy in dance survives in poetry and art, in present-day Central Asian folk dances, as well as practices in the *zurkhaneh* and in the Mevlevi *sema*, all of which share connections to Persian culture. Almost a thousand years after the demise of the Sogdians, yet another Silk Road dance form emerged, also characterized by dazzling spins.

## INDIAN DANCE IN CENTRAL ASIA

While commerce brought Central Asian dance to China, conquest brought Central Asians to Indian dance. The

Timurid conqueror Zahir-din-ud Mohammad Babur, a descendent of both Genghis Khan and Tamerlane, failed for many years to win back his hereditary capital of Samarkand. He finally turned his ambitions for empire south, moving into the Punjab in northern India to defeat the ruler Ibrahim Khan Lodi in 1526 at the Battle of Panipat. Fierce in battle, Babur was also a poet who built gardens and wrote the first autobiography in Islamic literature, the *Baburnama*. Babur cultivated a new political and cultural entity, the Mughal Dynasty, which ruled India from 1526 to 1858. Poets, architects, painters, musicians, craftsmen, and religious scholars, from all over the East found patronage at the Mughal court – and so did dancers. When Babur divvied up the spoils following the Battle of Panipat, he "gifted" each of his royal women "one special dancing-girl of the dancing-girls of Sultan Ibrahim, with one gold plate full of jewels."[18] At Babur's grand celebratory feast in 1528, local Indian acrobats identified as "*lulis*" performed and "many dancing girls also came and danced."[19]

In India, the Mughals encountered a dancescape rooted in Hinduism and based on the *Natya Shashtra*, a sacred Sanskrit treatise on the performing arts dating to 200 BCE or even earlier. It describes numerous facets of the performing arts, specific dance elements, and includes the concept of *rasa*, which emphasizes the goal of creating an emotion or sentiment capable of transporting audiences to a heightened consciousness, a level of greater spiritual awareness. The eight classical Indian dance forms – Odissi, Bharatanatyam, Kathakali, Mohiniyattam, Sattriya, Kuchipudi, Manipuri, and Kathak – all share roots in the *Natya Shastra*. However, Kathak, which developed under the Muslim Mughals, remains distinct.[20] The feet are not turned out or in deep bent knee positions; Kathak features a natural "straight leg." Kathak is the only Indian classical dance with fast, intricate spins – known as *chakkar* – that can be done rapidly in place and Kathak dancers, male and female alike, perform knee spins. Fast spins also occur in the Rajput *ghoomar* folk dance, so they may have entered the Kathak dance vocabulary in that way.[21] The unique qualities of Kathak reflect the blended nature of the Moghul court, "a synthesis of ethnic, cultural and political elements from India, Iran, and Central Asia."[22] In architecture, the iconic Taj Mahal symbolizes this cultural confluence. In dance, it is Kathak that embodies these legacies.

Accounts of the origin of Kathak point to the itinerant *kathakars* – or storytellers – who traveled with performances of tales from Hindu legends, using expressive gestures to convey these sacred stories. As divine storytellers, some dancers became attached to Hindu temples where they performed in the courtyards. The Mughals, as Sunni Muslims, considered Hindus and Sikhs as infidels, and viewed dance as entertainment rather than sacred worship, bringing it into the secular setting of the Moghul court.

Different levels of status distinguished female entertainers.[23] Some lived beyond the palace walls and could be hired for performances by nobles and other elites, while others only performed within the confines of the harem, entertaining other women and the emperor himself, along with his family members and high-ranking courtiers. Musicians occupied a low social status in traditional Islamic society and dancers ranked even lower, but through their beauty, skill, and charm these artists could enchant even the most powerful of men.[24] Dancers became essential entertainment at festive events like coronations and royal weddings, "signifiers of celebration and good fortune."[25]

One group of women had a unique status that allowed them to travel between these gendered worlds of the Moghul court. These were the courtesans, the *tawaifs*, who were well-educated in the arts of dance, music, and poetry. Sought after for their beauty and accomplishments, they formed alliances with men of power and wealth, managing to accumulate personal fortunes and enjoy some autonomy and prestige in a world where women had little control over their own fate.[26] The subject of the poetic *ghazals* that the *tawaif* performed in song and dance often expressed the *rasa* of *shringara*, the emotional state of attraction, of romantic and erotic love. As the Mughal empire grew in wealth and power, so did the prestige of the educated courtesans, trained in all the nuances of court etiquette. Some formed deep romantic relationships and were taken into royal harems. But the *tawaifs* also became the tragic heroines in cautionary tales about the power of seduction and inappropriate love.[27]

Lal Kunwar, an accomplished singer and dancer, captured the affection of Jahandar Shah so that he raised her to the status of a queen when he ascended the Moghul throne, though he reigned only a year before he was overthrown and murdered. Lal Kunwar spent her remaining days confined to the widow's quarters of the Red Fort in Delhi. Another tale, that of the dancer Anarkali ("pomegranate flower") and her ill-fated romance with Prince Salim, son of Emperor Akbar, seems to be merely legend. But whether Anarkali was entombed alive, escaped, or even actually existed, her story was immortalized centuries later in the 1960 Bollywood film *Moghul-e-Azzam* which depicted forbidden love against the backdrop of music and dance at the Mughal court.

The *tawaif* and their dance developed more fully around three *gharana* lineages – Lucknow, Jaipur, and Banaras. These schools developed different styles, with Lucknow and Banaras emphasizing *abhinaya* – the expressive, often gestural portion of the dance, intended to lead an audience toward the emotional state of *rasa* as defined in the *Natya Shastra*. The Jaipur *gharana* emphasized fast footwork, accented by the *gunghroo*, the small melodious bells tied around the ankles of the dancers.

## THE BRITISH IN INDIA

When the British arrived in India in 1608, it was initially for trade under the auspices of the East India Company, which raised and maintained its own army. The very same riches and resources that Babur had noted in his *Baburnama* also astounded the British. Some of these early merchants became fabulously rich and embraced Indian culture, even maintaining their own troupes of dancers and musicians to entertain their guests.[28] The British referred to what is now known as Kathak dance by the term *nautch*, an Anglicized form of the Hindi/Urdu word *nach*, meaning dance, but which came to be used to describe a dance party, as well as a performer of dance, "a nautch girl."

*Nautch* parties became grand entertainment for the civilians and soldiers of the East India Company, later performing for the British Army after the Crown seized control of India from the Company in 1857. When the Prince of Wales visited India, he was feted with a *nautch* performance. One Englishwoman who lived in Calcutta in the early 1800s, left a romantic description of a *nautch* party. The "glittering dresses of the dancing girls, their slow and graceful movement" combined with the luxurious setting, and the scent of the attar of roses and sandalwood incense, created the ambience of "some enchanted region...a fairy vision."[29] There were male dancers as well, "fine and tall young men attired in very rich costume" who performed dances similar to those of the nautch dancers, "with great agility and much grace."[30]

While the invading forces that established the Mughal empire had created a court culture that could patronize highly-skilled dancers, the incursion of the British Army fostered a climate that eventually led to the downfall of the *tawaifs*. These women, with their alluring dances about romantic love, performed with enticing facial expressions, fascinated the first Englishmen who came to India. But such open expressions of sexual desire played quite differently with some elements of Victorian-era Anglo culture. In 1858, the British classified the highly accomplished *tawaifs* in the same category as common prostitutes and increasingly subjected them to harsh colonial regulation and nationalist moral crusades. Missionaries and educated Indian social reformers joined forces in 1892 to launch the "anti-nautch" movement, labeling "nautch girls" as "public prostitutes." *Nautch* parties, they warned, should be boycotted because they "only give opportunities to the fallen women to beguile and tempt young men."[31] However, one opponent of the movement, Otto Rothfeld, in his work, *Women of India*, defended dance as "the most living and developed of Indian arts." He asserted that their dancing was "graceful and decorous, carefully draped and restrained" while admitting that the dancers "do not as a rule preserve that strict code of chastity which is extracted from the marrying women."[32]

As India struggled for independence from the British, there was a movement to reclaim the dance traditions that had suffered. Humiliated by the connection with prostitution, and the perceived abasement of Indian womanhood, dance specialists endeavored to cover up this "shameful" past, emphasizing the religious legacy of the *kathakars* instead of their link to Muslim Moghul court entertainers. Male teachers increasingly became the voices of authority on Kathak, advancing a standard history that outlined "a linear progression from temple to court to urban stage through the activities of male hereditary dancers."[33] They affirmed "the devotional and spiritual aspects of the dance" while diminishing the previous prominence of the *tawaifs* with their ambiguous moral and social status under Muslim overlords.[34] More recently the vital and active role of female dancers in shaping the development of Kathak has emerged through research by scholars who seek to spotlight a more prominent role for marginalized voices, specifically those of the *tawaif* who nurtured and performed the art.[35] No longer an entertainment for conquerors and their entourages, Kathak now enjoys global appreciation as a respected classical artform.

## BHANGRA AROUND THE WORLD

Less than a century after the death of the last Moghul emperor in 1862 and the decline of the *tawaif*, another Indian dance, *bhangra*, evolved from agrarian roots to eventually claim a place on the international stage. It began in the fertile Punjab, the "land of five rivers" known as India's breadbasket, a region conquered by the Moguls in 1526, annexed by the East India Company in 1849, and seized by the British Empire in 1858.

Bhangra began as a vigorous men's harvest dance, with motions connected to farming activities of plowing, sowing, and harvesting.[36] Specific to one area of the Punjab, Sialkot,[37] the dance was predominantly performed in the spring when crops like wheat and barley, planted in the cooler months of late autumn, became ripe for harvest. This coincided with the annual Sikh *Visakhi* festival which marked the beginning of the new year with religious observances and celebrations. The harvest brought income that could be spent at annual fairs, providing a welcome respite from labor.

In its original form, men gathered after the daily work of harvesting to dance bhangra. Characterized by jumping, squatting, leaping, with raised arms and lifted knees, the highly aerobic dance requires stamina and strength.[38] Participants danced vigorously in a circular path pausing as one person stood in the center to sing often erotic verses.[39] When signaled by a special cadence on the **dhol** – a double headed barrel drum central to bhangra – dancing resumed, a release of male energy connected to the *rasa* of *veer*, the signature mood of the male warrior.[40] Punjabi women had their own lively, hip-swinging dance, *giddah*, performed to similar rhythms but which men were not permitted to watch.

A communal, participatory activity, bhangra was not universal to the entire Punjab since each area within this large region had its own folk dance traditions. In 1947, the British Partition of India divided Punjab in two, with the Muslim majority in West Punjab assigned to Pakistan, and the Hindu majority in East Punjab becoming part of India. The Partition resulted in violence, death, and disruption; many fled their homes, ending up in refugee camps. In this national trauma, the Punjab Indian state lost more than half its land, but men continued to dance, even performing for Prime Minister Nehru in 1948, during his visit to a refugee camp.[41] The following year, a group of men displaced by the Partition created a bhangra team, beginning the transformation into a performance dance.

Newly decolonized India sought to define its identity, holding Independence Day celebrations and adopting a new national anthem and a new flag. Adjusting to change, some of the still existing princely states created the "Patiala and East Punjab States Union" (PEPSU) with the support of the Raja of Nalagarh who extended his royal patronage to the fledgling bhangra dance team in 1952, to represent PEPSU.[42] One dancer, Manohar Deepak, created a "judicious combination" by adding dance elements "from various places in Punjab."[43] When musicians and dancers from the itinerant Bazigar clan migrated from the Western Punjab, they shared their regional dances.

Invited by the Ministry of Defense to represent PEPSU for the Republic Day festivities in New Delhi, January 26, 1954, the dancers shared their Punjabi identity when various Indian states participated in a parade and performances with their distinctive music and dance. One observer noted that while other dances in the event had "far greater artistic value," bhangra won over the audience.

> The gentle opening followed by the triumphant, powerfully suggestive yells, seemed to fascinate the women. That these tall sinuous men could be as soft one minute and as strong the next seemed to stimulate them, as indeed is the whole purpose of the dance.[44]

This exuberant vigor of Punjabi bhangra embodied the energy of new India, making it an ideal national "calling card" for dance teams at international youth festivals that emerged in the wake of WWII.

Early in the development of the Indian film industry, that became known as Bollywood, bhangra dance episodes became popular, sometimes augmented with acrobatic elements which were absent from the original dance. Because films were a central form of shared entertainment throughout India, these Bollywood representations influenced perceptions and expectations of bhangra performances. Cinematic portrayals became so popular that from the early 1990s, bhangra became "the most widely utilized folk dance form in Bollywood," eventually moving it from its regional identity of Punjab "to become a key part of a 'national' popular culture."[45]

Punjabis embraced the dance as their specific identity marker. In place of the annual harvest fairs, Punjabi
youth gathered on the campuses of Indian universities like
Mohindra College in Patiala. A hereditary *dhol* player from
the Bazigar community, Bhana Ram, trained the Mohindra
College team, selecting dancers based on height and chest
size, creating a formidable appearance on stage.[46]

No longer a participatory folk dance, bhangra evolved into
a well-rehearsed, synchronized performance with structured
choreographies, sometimes under the direction of a dance
coach. Instead of absorbing the dance in the original village
context, Punjabi university students learned and performed
a new kind of bhangra, an "invented tradition," including
movements gleaned from other Punjabi folk dances.[47]

The end of rule by the British Raj in 1947 brought opportunities for Punjabi emigration to the United Kingdom.
The children of these émigrés sought places where they
could safely gather with other young South Asians, as well
as escape their parents' watchful eyes. Girls were especially
under scrutiny, forbidden any unchaperoned activity after
dark. The youth organized secret afternoon bhangra parties where boys and girls could meet and dance; traditional
Punjabi music morphed in the hands of popular "desi DJs"
who blended traditional songs and rhythms with Western
genres like rap, reggae, and house creating a new "British
bhangra" music.[48] Lyrics changed to include themes of
communal identity, politics, and issues relevant to the lives
of diasporic Punjabis as well as a "longing for the 'homeland.'"[49] Punjabi women growing up in UK culture, started
to challenge the traditional gender roles of Punjabi/Sikh
culture embedded in bhangra music and dance environments. Female bhangra DJs like Radical Sista in Britain,
Rekha in New York, and Ameeta in Canada challenged
the gendered norms of Punjabi traditions. Parv Kaur created
her *dhol* band "Eternal Taal," proving that women had the
strength and stamina to play the large barrel drum, carried
by a strap across the body.[50] More recently, the first female
Asian rapper, Hard Kaur, defied patriarchal gender hierarchies and misogyny.[51]

Changes in the 1965 U.S. immigration law abolished *de facto* discrimination against Asians and Punjabis were among the first Indians to relocate to the U.S., bringing their music and dance with them. Just as bhangra groups had formed at universities in India, Punjabi student associations began to take root on U.S. and Canadian campuses with membership including other Indians and South Asians. These bhangra performances appealed to many diasporic Indians who faced both "detachment from the homeland and longing for the idea of a lost cultural heritage."[52]

In 1993, the South Asian Society of George Washington University hosted Bhangra Blowout, the first intercollegiate competition in the U.S., growing from a modest event to sell-out performances in large auditoriums. Other colleges followed and female students began to cross the traditional gender boundaries to join all-male groups. Competition judges, usually drawn from an older generation, bristled at the addition of females performing bhangra which challenged the prohibition against women dancing in public.

Bhangra teams, some co-ed, prepared elaborate, high-energy choreographies with constantly shifting floor patterns set to a medley of songs, both traditional and hybrid club versions. They incorporated traditional objects into the dance, such as the *sapp*, a sort of wooden lattice clapper that expands and contracts, and the *khund*, a farmer's staff.[53] As dance competitions grew increasingly intricate, some teams included sensational elements such as special lighting effects and acrobatic feats. Costuming became brighter and more resplendent than the original rustic farmer attire. Male and female dancers, often paired in matching colors, added another visual element to the formations when they parted and merged at different points in the choreography. The men's tall, distinctive turbans made them imposing figures on stage, a powerful presence that has become an iconic image of Indian dance.

All-female bhangra teams have emerged, in spite of discouragement from competition judges who told them that they "shouldn't be doing this."[54] In 2019, the all-women

DC Bhangra Crew (DCBC) hosted _Raniyaan di Raunaq_, America's first all-women bhangra competition.[55] One dancer explained the appeal of bhangra over the traditionally feminine _giddha_ as "more empowering .... because it is stronger. I can stand with my feet wider. I can make powerful movements...."[56] Another participant suggested that because bhangra is "very much a man's dance" the movements "make women feel strong." She explained, "I get a high off their strength. It's so manly. I absolutely love it. I want to copy it."[57]

The valiant warrior energy of _veer rasa_, embodied in bhangra, may explain its appeal in times of trial. Canadian dancer Gurdeep Pandher celebrated on video after he received his COVID-19 vaccine by going to a frozen lake in Yukon to "dance Bhangra on it for joy" in a spirit of "hope and positivity... for everyone's health and well-being." Pandher explained that bhangra, part of his heritage, "is a dance that still keeps me happy and vibrant."[58]

In a little more than one hundred years, bhangra evolved from a village dance, to a national stage dance, to a diaspora heritage dance,[59] to a dance of female empowerment. Now with a global following, bhangra's popularity extends beyond those of South Asian heritage.

Separated by over a thousand years, three dances of differing origins intertwined with the fates of empires, one embraced as an "exotic" diversion in T'ang China, another developed as refined entertainment at the Moghul court, and a third became an embodied symbol of national vitality for independent India. The decline of T'ang imperial power and changing attitudes toward foreigners lessened the Sogdian presence in China but the spinning dance technique surfaces in still-existing traditions with connections to Persian culture. Moghul patronage pulled an Indian devotional dance into an Indo-Persian-Turkic court culture where it developed into a brilliant, sophisticated art, only to suffer debasement under the British Raj. Restored and rehabilitated by Indian dance masters, Kathak found new appreciative audiences beyond the elite. Finally, a vigorous village dance done to celebrate harvest provided a source of pride and endurance for displaced populations from a divided homeland. Providing vitality and strength for national identity, at home and abroad, women also have embraced bhangra's embodied power as an affirmation of equality.

Empires collapse, civilizations crumble, but dance continues to travel within the human body as intangible heritage. Ever resilient, dance evolves with changing needs and contexts. Beauty and strength continue to captivate, even attracting those outside of the cultures of origin to give dance a home in their own foreign bodies. From these ever-unfolding adoptions and adaptations, a heightened cultural sensitivity may emerge.

# FURTHER READING

Ballantyne, Tony. *Between Colonialism and Diaspora: Sikh Cultural Formations in an Imperial World.* Durham: Duke University Press, 2006. Ballantyne traces the remarkable journey of a village harvest dance that became a transnational symbol of Sikh identity and a powerful testimony of resilience.

Chakravorty, Pallabi. *Bells of Change: Kathak Dance, Women, and Modernity in India.* Kolkata: Seagull Books, 2008. The author, a South Asian feminist with a doctorate in anthropology, offers a fresh investigation into the origins and development of Kathak that highlights the marginalized voices of women.

Hansen, Valerie. *The Silk Road: A New History.* Oxford: Oxford University Press, 2012. This innovative approach uses archeological evidence to replace the romanticized Silk Road with a reality evidenced by physical objects that tell cultural, social, and economic stories of cross-cultural exchange. Hansen focuses on seven important trade centers, illustrating her findings with vivid color plates.

Walker, Margaret E. *India's Kathak Dance in Historical Perspective.* Farnham, England: Ashgate, 2014. The author investigates accepted origin stories of Kathak to reveal a complex and fascinating history of a dance form that endured colonialism and post-colonial backlash to become global performance art.

Witbeck, Quisqueya G. "Breaking Boundaries: Bhangra as a Mechanism for Identity Formation and Sociopolitical Refuge Among South Asian American Youths". ProQuest Dissertations

Publishing, 2018. This dissertation reveals the profound and positive impact of a folk dance on minority youth in their search for identity.

## TIMELINE

500–800 CE – Sogdian trade with China peaks, trading luxuries, such as gemstones, horses, grape wine, precious metals, amber, furs, slaves, and foreign dancers.

755–763 CE – Rebellion of the General An Lushan results in foreigners and foreign ideas becoming regarded with suspicion.

1526–1858 – The Mughal Dynasty values poets, architects, painters, musicians, craftsmen, religious scholars, and dancers.

1608 – British arrive in India.

1857 – The British Crown seizes control of India.

January 26, 1954 – Dancers represent PEPSU to perform for the Republic Day festivities in New Delhi.

1965 – U.S. immigration law abolishes *de facto* discrimination against Asians, causing many Punjabis to move to the U.S.

## BIBLIOGRAPHY

Agrawal, Nadya. "This All-Girl Punjabi Dance Team is Crushing Their Male Competitors." Vice. April 24, 2016. www.vice.com/en/article/wnwv89/this-all-girl-punjabi-dance-team-is-crushing-their-male-competitors.

Ballantyne, Tony. "Displacement, Diaspora, and Difference in the Making of Bhangra." In *Between Colonialism and Diaspora: Sikh Cultural Formations in an Imperial World*, edited by Tony Ballantyne, 121–159. Durham: Duke University Press.

Beauchamp, Fay. "Tang Dynasty Revolution and Poetry: Bai Juyi's 'Construction' of Yang Guifei." *History, Literature, and the Construction of "Memory" in Asia*, no. 14:1 (2009): 37.

Beveridge, Annette Susannah. *Babur Nama*, Trans. London: Penguin Books, 2006.

Chacko, Elizabeth and Rajiv Menon, "Longings and belongings: Indian American youth identity, folk dance competitions, and the construction of 'tradition'." *Ethnic and Racial Studies* 36, no. 1 (2013): 103.

Chamnet, Lee. "The An Shi Rebellion and Rejection of the Other in Tang China, 618–763." Master's Thesis. University of Alberta, 2012.

Dhurandhar, Sunita. "Return to Bhangra: from dance clubs to gym clubs, young South Asian women reclaim a dance never meant for them." *Colorlines Magazine*. June 22, 2005. www.thefreelibrary.com/eturn+to+Bhangra%3A+from+dance+clubs+to+gym+clubs%2C+young+South+Asian...-a0133188357.

Gray, Laurel Victoria. "*Tanoura* is Sleeping: Exploring an Ancient Whirling Ritual in Cairo." *Habibi* 18, no. 2, (2000): 20–27. http://thebestofhabibi.com/volume-18-no-2-september-2000/tanoura/.

___. "Wizards and Harlots: The Tainted Status of Musicians and Dancers within the Islamic Context." *Habibi* 19, no. 2, 40–45.

Hansen, Valerie. *The Silk Road: A New History*. Oxford University Press, Oxford, 2012.

Joncheere, Ayla. "Kalbeliya Dance from Rajasthan: Invented Gypsy Form or Traditional Snake Charmers' Folk Dance?" *Dance Research Journal* 49, no. 1 (2017): 42. DOI:10.1017/S0149767717000055.

Kishore, Vikrant. "Representations of Indian Folk Dance Forms in the Song and Dance Sequences of Contemporary Bollywood Cinema." Doctoral dissertation. Royal Melbourne Institute of Technology, 2010.

Laufer, Berthold. *Sino-Iranica: Chinese Contributions to the History of Civilization in Ancient Iran, with Special Reference to the History of Cultivated Plants and Products*. United States: Field Museum of Natural History, 1919.

Leslie, Donald Daniel. "Persian Temples in T'ang China." *Monumenta Serica* 35 (1981): 278. Accessed September 26, 2020. www.jstor.org/stable/40726510.

Mair, Victor H. ed., trans. *The Shorter Columbia Anthology of Traditional Chinese Literature*. (New York: Columbia University Press, 2001), 149–150.

Nevile, Pran. *Nautch Girls of the Raj*. Penguin Books, London, 2009.

Pandher, Gurdeep. "'Things are going to be great': Whitehorse Bhangra dancer celebrates his COVID-19 vaccine," *As It Happens*. CBC. March 2, 2021. www.cbc.ca/radio/asithappens/as-it-happens-the-tuesday-edition-1.5933726/things-are-going-to-be-great-whitehorse-bhangra-dancer-celebrates-his-covid-19-vaccine-1.5933727.

Roy, Anjali Gera. "Gendering Dance." *Religions*. Basel, 11, no. 4, (2020): 202. DOI:10.3390/rel11040202.

Schafer, Edward H. *The Golden Peaches of Samarkand: A Study of T'ang Exotics*. University of California Press, 1963/1985.

Schofield, Katherine Butler. "The Courtesan Tale: Female Musicians and Dancers in Mughal Historical Chronicles, c.1556–1748." *Gender & History* 24, no. 1 (2012): 150–171.

Schreffler, Gibb. "Situating bhangra dance: a critical introduction." *South Asian History and Culture*, 4:3, (2013): 384–412. DOI: 10.1080/19472498.2013.808514.

Sinnenberg, Jackson, "*Raniyaan di Raunaq*, America's first all-women's bhangra competition, shakes up the status quo." *Washington Post Express.* August 8, 2019. www.washingtonpost. com/express/2019/08/08/raniyaan-di-raunaq-americas-first-all-womens-bhangra-competition-shakes-up-status-quo/.

Vishal, Mundra "Obesity management: Dancing to the Bhangra beat." *Indian Journal of Endocrinology and Metabolism*2012 Sep–Oct; 16(5): 868–869. www.ncbi.nlm.nih.gov/pmc/articles/PMC3475935/.

Walker, Margaret E. "The 'Nautch' Reclaimed: Women's Performance Practice in Nineteenth-Century North India." *South Asia: Journal of South Asian Studies* 37:4, (2014): 551–567. DOI: 10.1080/00856401.2014.938714.

Wade, Bonnie C. *Imaging Sound: An Ethnomusicological Study of Music, Art, and Culture in Mughal.* University of Chicago, 1998.

Wen, Xin. "What's in a Surname? Central Asian Participation in the Culture of Naming of Medieval China." *Tang Studies* 34:1 (2016): 88.

# NOTES

1 These caravan routes date back to at least the 2nd century BCE, but it was not until 1877, that the German geographer Ferdinand von Richthofen coined the term "silk road" (*seiden-strasse*). See Scott C. Levi, "Silk Roads, Real and Imagined," *The Bukharan Crisis* (University of Pittsburgh Press, 2020), 37–69.

2 Valerie Hansen, *The Silk Road: A New History* (Oxford: Oxford University Press, 2012), 4.

3 Donald Daniel Leslie, "Persian Temples in T'ang China," *Monumenta Serica* 35 (1981): 278. Accessed September 26, 2020, www.jstor.org/stable/40726510.

4 Xin Wen, "What's in a Surname? Central Asian Participation in the Culture of Naming of Medieval China," *Tang Studies*, 34(1), (2016): 88.

5 T'ang Annuals cited in Berthold Laufer, *Sino-Iranica: Chinese Contributions to the History of Civilization in Ancient Iran, with Special Reference to the History of Cultivated Plants and Products, Volume 15, Issue 3. Publication Series.* Volume 15. (1919), Field Museum of Natural History, p. 494.

6 Edward H. Schafer, *The Golden Peaches of Samarkand: A Study of T'ang Exotics,* University of California Press, 1962, p. 55.

7 Bai Juyi, cited in Schafer.

8 Schafer, p. 56.

9  Bai Juyi, cited by Schafer, 55.

10  Hansen, 144.

11  Bai Juyi translated by Victor H. Mair, ed., trans. *The Shorter Columbia Anthology of Traditional Chinese Literature* (New York: Columbia University Press, 2001), 149–150.

12  T'ang Annuals cited by Schafer, 56.

13  Bai Juyi, cited in Mair.

14  Fay Beauchamp, "Tang Dynasty Revolution and Poetry: Bai Juyi's 'Construction' of Yang Guifei," *History, Literature, and the Construction of "Memory" in Asia*, no. 14:1, (2009): 37.

15  Lee Chamnet, "The An Shi Rebellion and Rejection of the Other in Tang China, 618–763," Master's Thesis, University of Alberta, 2012.

16  Chamnet questions the figure of 36 million since the rebellion dislocated populations and disrupted census accuracy.

17  Laurel Victoria Gray, "*Tanoura* is Sleeping: Exploring an Ancient Whirling Ritual in Cairo," *Habibi* 18, no. 2, (2000): 20–27, http://thebestofhabibi.com/volume-18-no-2-september-2000/tanoura/.

18  *Humayannam* of Gulabadon Begum, cited by Bonnie C. Wade in *Imagining Sound: An Ethnomusicological Study of Music, Art, and Culture in Mughal India*, University of Chicago Press, Chicago, 1998, 84.

19  *Babur Nama*, Annette Susannah Beveridge, trans., Penguin Books, London, 2006, 324–325.

20  According to Margaret Walker, "nowhere in the indigenous or colonial literature before 1900 is the dance art of women performers called *kathak*." Margaret E. Walker "The 'Nautch' Reclaimed: Women's Performance Practice in Nineteenth-Century North India," *South Asia: Journal of South Asian Studies*, 37:4, (2014): 553. DOI: 10.1080/00856401.2014.938714.

21  Ayla Joncheere, "Kalbeliya Dance from Rajasthan: Invented Gypsy Form or Traditional Snake Charmers' Folk Dance?" *Dance Research Journal*, 49, no. 1 (2017): 42. DOI:10.1017/S0149767717000055.

22  Katherine Butler Schofield, "The Courtesan Tale: Female Musicians and Dancers in Mughal Historical Chronicles, c.1556–1748," *Gender & History* 24, no. 1 (2012): 151. https://doiorg.proxygw.wrlc.org/10.1111/j.1468-0424.2011.01673.x.

23  Schofield, 152–158.

24  Laurel Victoria Gray, "Wizards and Harlots: The Tainted Status of Musicians and Dancers within the Islamic Context," *Habibi* 19, no. 2, 40– 45.

25  Schofield, 153.

26  For the period 1858–1877, "courtesans in Lucknow belonged to the highest income bracket and possessed substantial property, political influence and cultural prestige." Cited in Schofield, 150.

27 Schofield, pp. 8–11.

28 Pran Nevile, *Nautch Girls of the Raj*, Penguin Books, London, 2009, 27.

29 Mrs S.C. Belnos, cited by Nevile, 36.

30 Nevile, 44.

31 Anti-nautch circular of 1893, cited in Nevile, 116.

32 Otto Rothfield, *Women of India* (London, 1920) cited in Nevile, 122.

33 Margaret Walker, Review of *Bells of Change: Kathak Dance, Women And Modernity In India,*
    *Dance Research Journal* A3 / 1 (2011): 105. https://doi.org/10.5406/danceresearchj.43.1.0105.

34 Margaret E. Walker, "The 'Nautch' Reclaimed: Women's Performance Practice in Nineteenth-Century North India," *South Asia: Journal of South Asian Studies*, 37:4, 551–567, (2014). DOI: 10.1080/00856401.2014.938714.

35 Walker, Review of *Bells Of Change*, 106; Walker, 552.

36 Gurdeep Pandher, "'Things are going to be great': Whitehorse Bhangra dancer celebrates his COVID-19 vaccine," *As It Happens*, CBC, March 2, 2021, www.cbc.ca/radio/asithappens/as-it-happens-the-tuesday-edition-1.5933726/things-are-going-to-be-great-whitehorse-bhangra-dancer-celebrates-his-covid-19-vaccine-1.5933727.

37 Gibb Schreffler, "Situating bhangra dance: a critical introduction," South Asian History and Culture, 4:3, (2013): 390. DOI: 10.1080/19472498.2013.808514.

38 Mundra Vishal suggests that the vigorous aerobic quality of bhangra, "may turn out to be the magic wand which can arrest the spread of obesity" in Vishal's article in "Obesity management: Dancing to the Bhangra beat," Indian Journal of Endocrinology and Metabolism, 2012 Sep–Oct; 16(5): 868–869.
    www.ncbi.nlm.nih.gov/pmc/articles/PMC3475935/.

39 Schreffler, 392.

40 Anjali Gera Roy, "Gendering Dance," *Religions*, Basel, 11, no. 4, (2020): 202. DOI:10.3390/rel11040202.

41 Schreffler, 394.

42 Schreffler, 395.

43 Manohar Deepak cited by Schreffler, 395.

44 Prakash Tandon in *Punjabi Century 1857–1947*, cited by Schreffler, 397.

45 Vikrant Kishore, "Representations of Indian Folk Dance Forms in the Song and Dance Sequences of Contemporary Bollywood Cinema," doctoral dissertation, Royal Melbourne Institute of Technology (2010): 205.

46 Anjali Gera Roy, "Gendering Dance," *Religions* 11, no. 4, (2020): 2. http://proxygw.wrlc.org/login?url=https://www-proquest-com.proxygw.wrlc.org/scholarly-journals/gendering-dance/docview/2393271881/se-2?accountid=11243.

47 Schreffler, 399.

48 Elizabeth Chacko and Rajiv Menon, "Longings and belong-ings: Indian American youth identity, folk dance competitions, and the construction of 'tradition'," *Ethnic and Racial Studies* 36, no. 1 (2013): 103.

49 Ibid.

50 Roy, 9.

51 Roy, 10.

52 Chacko, 98.

53 Schreffler, 77.

54 Nadya Agrawal, "This All-Girl Punjabi Dance Team is Crushing Their Male Competitors," Vice, April 24, 2016, www.vice.com/en/article/wnwv89/this-all-girl-punjabi-dance-team-is-crushing-their-male-competitors.

55 Jackson Sinnenberg, "*Raniyaan di Raunaq,* America's first all-women's bhangra competition, shakes up the status quo," *Washington Post Express,* August 8, 2019. www.washingtonpost.com/express/2019/08/08/raniyaan-di-raunaq-americas-first-all-womens-bhangra-competition-shakes-up-status-quo/.

56 Shyamala Moorty quoted by Sunita Dhurandhar, "Return to Bhangra: from dance clubs to gym clubs, young South Asian women reclaim a dance never meant for them," *Colorlines Magazine,* June 22, 2005, www.thefreelibrary.com/eturn+to+Bhangra%3A+from+dance+clubs+to+gym+clubs%2C+young+South+Asian...-a0133188357.

57 Sarina Jain quoted by Dhurandhar, op.cit.

58 Gurdeep Pandher interview, "'Things are going to be great': Whitehorse Bhangra dancer celebrates his COVID-19 vaccine," *As It Happens,* CBC, March 2, 2021, www.cbc.ca/radio/asithappens/as-it-happens-the-tuesday-edition-1.5933726/things-are-going-to-be-great-whitehorse-bhangra-dancer-celebrates-his-covid-19-vaccine-1.5933727.

59 Schreffler, 385.

# CHAPTER 3

# *Asé!* in Action
## Dance in the American African Diaspora

*Joanna Dee Das*

People gather in a circle around two men who face each other, knees bent, weight shifted forward over the balls of their feet, bouncing to the rhythm, ready to spring into action. A break in the percussive music signals *go*. One man jumps off both feet and kicks his left leg high while the other drops down, knees bending deeply. The man on the ground rises up, then lowers again when his opponent circles a leg over him. He pulses in this deep knee bend, hands on the ground for support, then stands. The two dancers step to the beat as they adjust their positions in the circle, reestablishing their spatial relationship and setting up for the next percussive attack.[1]

When offered such a description, my U.S. American college students in 2022 might guess that I am describing a hip hop battle between two breakers, although high kicks from a standing position are not generally a part of the repertoire. Some, with more knowledge of dance outside their own national context, might recognize elements of Brazilian *capoeira*.[2] Certainly none will guess **ladja** from Martinique (also known as *danmyé* in the northern part of the island), a form that has not reached the same level of global circulation as the other two. If I add layers of specificity, the distinction of ladja begins to emerge. The participants in this film clip from 1936 wear collared button-down shirts, dress pants, and hats. A *bèlè* drum, in which the musician uses his foot to change the pitch, guides the dancers. Most importantly, the location of this *won* (circle) embeds ladja in local Martinican

DOI: 10.4324/9781003185918-3

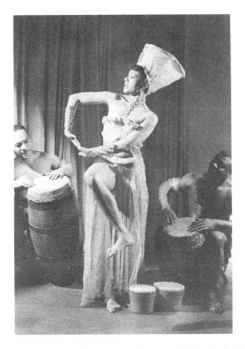

**Figure 3.1:** Katherine Dunham in *Cabin in the Sky*, 1940.
Photographer: Bob Golby.
Source: Courtesy of Special Collections Research Center, Morris Library,
Southern Illinois University Carbondale.

histories. Nonetheless, undeniable commonalities, both aesthetic and philosophical, link ladja to capoeira and breaking.
A circle of energy coheres those watching and those dancing
into a collective. The movement is in intimate conversation
with the music. The intent is not to harm, but to demonstrate skill and embodied cleverness in negotiating conflict.
Finally, the people who created the dances were of African
descent living in the Americas, or, what one could call the
American African Diaspora.[3]

What is the African Diaspora? The term first appeared in the
1960s to describe a phenomenon that had begun centuries
earlier. In its primary definition, a diaspora is a scattering of a
people from a homeland, often but not exclusively through

forced migration. For many years, the African Diaspora was imagined as a concrete place: a connected web of communities of people of African descent, radiating out from West and Central Africa to the Americas along the lines of the trans-Atlantic slave trade, also known as **the Middle Passage**, that began in the 16th century and lasted until the mid-19th century. The African Diaspora is now imagined globally, with reach into Europe, Asia, and everywhere that people of African descent have migrated. Its temporal dimensions have stretched to include migrations both before and after the centuries of the slave trade. Furthermore, cultural theorists such as Stuart Hall, Paul Gilroy, and Brent Hayes Edwards have disrupted the sense of fixed positions, instead positing that diaspora is consciously made and remade, the connections forged through intentional effort.[4]

One of the connectivities of diaspora is dance, an art form that communicates embodied meaning through time and across space. Virtually no dance created in the Americas from the 16th century onwards has remained untouched by Africanist influence, not just dances like ladja but also ones often thought of as European or "Latin," such as ballet or the Argentine tango. I utilize "Africanist" after Brenda Dixon Gottschild, who writes that the term "denotes concepts and practices that exist in Africa and the African diaspora and have their sources in concepts or practices from Africa."[5] Gottschild is one of the scholars who has attempted to provide a broad analytical framework to interpret such a wide range of dance practices. In 1966, art historian Robert Farris Thompson wrote a highly influential essay: "An Aesthetic of the Cool: West African Dance." In it, he outlined five qualities of West African dance that he believed manifested in diasporic forms as well: the dominance of percussion; multiple meter (meaning, multiple rhythms happening at the same time); **apart dancing**; call-and-response; and dance as moral system, with a final assessment of West African dance as possessing an overall "aesthetic of the cool."[6] Two years later, Jean and Marshall Stearns developed their own list of Africanist influences that they saw in U.S. jazz dance: the whole foot on the ground; movement from a bent knees position; imitation of animals; improvisation; **centrifugal**

**movement** from the hips and pelvis; and performed to "propulsive rhythm."[7]

While stressing the "enormous complexity" of the dance forms of the hundreds of millions of people of African descent around the globe, Kariamu Welsh Asante's "Commonalities in African Dance: An Aesthetic Foundation" (1985), like Thompson's essay, laid out a set of seven principles, which she called "senses," of African dance: polyrhythm (akin to multiple meter), polycentrism (having multiple centers of movement in the body), curvilinearity (emphasis on circles and curves), dimensionality (that music, dance, and other arts are richly textured and layered and include dimensions beyond those that can be measured), epic memory (drawing on a spiritual and ancestral sense of memory), holism (emphasizing the whole rather than the individual), and repetition, which is not just repeating something exactly the same way, but with increasing intensity.[8] Continuing in this vein, in 1996 Brenda Dixon Gottschild outlined "First Premises of an Africanist Aesthetic" that included valuing process; an emphasis on movement even in written or spoken texts; embracing the conflict, polycentrism/polyrhythm, high-affect juxtaposition (dynamic contrasts that create surprise, irony, or comedy), ephebism (power, vitality, and attack), and, in reference to Thompson, "the aesthetic of the cool."[9]

These treatises on Africanist aesthetics have been highly useful to challenge Eurocentric vocabularies and mindsets about dance. At the same time, there are limitations. Sometimes lists lead students to think that Africanist aesthetics have not changed in 400 years. Recent research counters such a static perspective, such as writing by Ana Paula Höfling on staging capoeira, my own about African performers at the 1893 World's Fair, and a recent volume edited by Kariamu Welsh, Esailama G.A. Diouf, and Yvonne Daniel that examines West African dancers in the United States in the 20th and 21st centuries.[10] African influence is dynamic and shifting. These lists can also limit how students understand the myriad contributions of people of African descent in the Americas outside of movements that register as "Africanist" based on the aforementioned qualities. As Nadine George-Graves asks, "Who are the identity watchdogs that determine whether or not a given set of identities in aggregate is significantly diasporic?"[11] It is not only Africanist aesthetics that have indelibly shaped dance in the Americas, but also the creative practices of Black people as they innovated in new contexts.

Thus, the term Black dance is also a useful analytic to bring into the conversation. Thomas DeFrantz and Anita Gonzalez identify two foundations of Black performance: the "manifestation of Africanist aesthetics" and "a response to histories that extend beyond Africa and its aesthetics."[12] Takiyah Nur Amin consolidates these two aspects in defining Black dance as "the multiple movement idioms that both originate within Black African culture and those that emerge as they are filtered through the experiences of Black people as a result of assimilating various cultural influences."[13] DeFrantz, in another essay titled "What Is Black Dance? What Can It Do?" invites readers to consider Black dance as "approaches to moving" rather than focus on specific steps. He writes that "Black performance exists to confirm the presence of Black people in the world," creating "possibilities for group communion." Black performance is an "aesthetic and social confirmation of a possibility of Black life" in the face of "disavowal, coercion and genocide."[14] Building upon such work, this chapter will discuss three case studies—the religious dances of Haitian Vodou, the theatrical dance of Katherine Dunham, and the social practice of hip hop—as windows into the ways one can approach thinking about dance in the African Diaspora. While I make a distinction between religious, theatrical, and social dance practices, the boundaries are porous. We cannot pin culture down; we must dance with it, following its flows and shifts.

The dances of Vodou have disseminated into many realms. Vodou as a religious practice developed in the 17th century among Africans living in Saint-Domingue, the French colony on the island of Hispaniola. Vodou dancers theorized and enacted the aesthetic, spiritual, ancestral, and political possibilities of their embodied expressions. Through danced religious ritual, practitioners simultaneously maintained ancestral connections to *Nan Guinée*, or African homeland, and responded to the brutal conditions of enslavement under French colonialism. The religious practice incorporates traditions from Fon, Yoruban, Ibo, Angolan, and other ethnic groups as well as from Catholicism. It emphasizes serving the spirits (*sevi loa*) as a way to communicate with the divine, with an ethos of reciprocity as the foundation. According to multiple sources, in August 1791, enslaved Africans gathered in Bois Caïman, a region in the north of the island, to prepare to revolt against the French. A Vodou ceremony, with music and dance, was an integral part. Even though the historical details about the August 1791 ceremony are unclear, the belief endured that Vodou created the solidarity necessary to overthrow one of the world's most powerful colonial empires. In 1939, Aimé Césaire famously wrote that Haiti was where *négritude*, or a Black consciousness, "first stood up."[15]

After the Revolution ended in 1804, with Haiti as the hemisphere's first Black republic, Vodou localized, as practitioners in small villages or family compounds (*lakous*) developed practices to serve their specific needs. Despite such variation, there are some commonalities that developed across ceremonies. One usually calls upon the loa Legba to open the gates, allowing the crossover between the spirit world and the human world; then there are various methods to call the spirits in, including the drawing of *vévés*, shaking of the *assons*, and drumming. But the way the spirit fully manifests is through dance, in which a loa "mounts" the devotee to communicate with the gathered practitioners. In the *yanvalou*, the dance of the loa Damballah, practitioners undulate the full extent of their spines, rippling like a wave, "drawing energy from the ground into bent knees, through the pelvis, up the back, into the chest, through the neck, and through the arms and fingertips."[16] For some the movement signifies reaching back across the ocean to Africa to connect with ancestors, and others embody it as calming prayer that relieves emotional distress by opening oneself up to a higher power. Those two aspects of ancestor and spirit are intertwined.[17]

Political and religious forces conspired to repress Vodou starting in the 19th century. In Haiti as elsewhere in the

Americas, elite classes attempted to erase Africanist cultural influence as a way to maintain white supremacist structures. In the United States, some claimed that the brutality of the Middle Passage, the fact that dozens of different ethnic groups from different parts of Africa mixed in their new locations, and the forced conversion to Christianity had destroyed African culture. This "myth," wrote anthropologist Melville Herskovits in 1941, "was one of the principle supports of race prejudice."[18] In Haiti, the ruling *mulatre* (mixed-race) class esteemed French culture above all else and enacted laws to ban not only Vodou rituals but also popular dances of the working class.[19]

In the midst of the US Occupation of Haiti from 1915 to 1934, Haitian intellectuals began to counter such violent repressions with the *indigénisme* movement. Anthropologist Jean Price-Mars argued that elite Haitians, who had focused on French culture, should instead embrace African heritage to gather the strength to resist the United States.[20] *Indigénisme* was tied to the internationalist New Negro Movement of the 1920s in which artists and intellectuals were beginning to recognize the relationship between Africanist cultural practices and the politics of resistance. In 1925, Arturo Schomburg famously told Black Americans to "dig up [their] past" in order to create a more just and equitable world; Nicolas Guillén, Fernando Ortiz, and others led the **Afrocubanismo movement** in Cuba.[21]

Inspired in part by American choreographer Katherine Dunham, about whom we will learn more later on, in the 1940s the Haitian government began to promote "folkloric" dance, which took the movements of Vodou and stripped them of their political and religious meanings. Those dancing Haitian folklore in state-sponsored schools and troupes were largely not the rural, working-class practitioners of Vodou, but the children of urban elites. Throughout the second half of the 20th century, Vodou dance diffused into multiple performance contexts: official government-sanctioned performances at the Bureau of Ethnology and international festivals; tourist shows at hotels that promised European and white American travelers an exotic Vodou ceremony experience; and international theatrical stages in the choreographic works of choreographer Jean-León Destiné and others.[22]

In the 21st century, Vodou still operates on multiple registers. It is still a religious practice for many Haitians and also choreographic inspiration for artists such as Jeanguy Saintus. Saintus, born in Haiti, trained with renowned master dancers such as Viviane Gauthier and Régine Montrosier Trouillot in folkloric, modern, and balletic idioms. He founded Ayikodans, a school and dance company, in 1987. His choreography pushes against expectations, both those who wish to see exoticism in his work and others who want him to conform to Eurocentric ideas of contemporary dance. He notes when certain conventions named as "contemporary," such as "fall and recover," are actually present in Vodou. When you feel the "trance" of possession approaching, he explains, you "go into that fall and rebound process."[23] Saintus also explores themes of queer desire through an approach scholar Mario LaMothe calls *dedouble*, or "the Haitian body desiring to unbind itself from prescriptions (fixed time, place, and socio-cultural conventions)." Saintus' work has been seen around the world, including in a 2019 production of *The Rite of Spring* for the River Phoenix Dance Company in the United Kingdom.[24]

One of the primary catalysts for the translation of Vodou to the concert dance stage was Katherine Dunham. Born in 1909 in a suburb of Chicago, Illinois, Dunham had loved to dance as a child but found few opportunities to pursue her passion until she moved to the city to attend the University of Chicago. Through connections she made at her older brother's theater troupe, Dunham began to take ballet and modern dance classes and co-founded multiple dance troupes, first the Ballet Nègre with Mark Turbyfill and then the Negro Dance Group with Ludmilla Speranzeva. But she felt something was missing – a depth of understanding of the Africanist cultural practices she was presenting onstage. To learn more, she turned to the field of anthropology. Dunham traveled to the Caribbean in 1935 under the auspices of a Rosenwald Fellowship to conduct research in Jamaica, Martinique, Trinidad, and most importantly, Haiti. Over the course of ten months, she not only learned new dance steps, but also absorbed *indigénisme* philosophy in Haiti. To paraphrase DeFrantz, she began to understand dance as a collective affirmation of Black life. She started her field research by looking for Africanist retentions, but instead developed a more nuanced understanding of cultural transformation in the inherently contemporary practices of her interlocutors. When Dunham returned to the United States in 1936, she established her own troupe that quickly became regarded as one of the top dance companies in the nation and eventually the world. Her new movement vocabulary incorporated multiple Afro-Caribbean forms, and she was unafraid to put Africanist aesthetics and practices front and center in her choreography. After attending Dunham's 1940 show *Tropics and Le Jazz "Hot"* in New York, Elie Lescot, Haitian ambassador to the United States, praised her for paving the way for Vodou rituals to find "a permanent niche in the temple of Terpsichorean Art." A year later when he became President of Haiti, Lescot insisted that a Haitian student group performing for a Folklore Congress in Washington include dance in its production.[25]

The dance *Shango* is an example of the new emphasis on Africanist aesthetics Dunham brought to the stage. Shango is the West African Yoruban god of fire, lightning, and thunder, and is also the name for the Orisha religious tradition of Trinidad. Dunham premiered the piece as a part of her Broadway show *Carib Song* (1945), which told the story of a Trinidadian fisherman and his unfaithful wife; *Shango* closes the first act. The piece begins with villagers gathering to make an offering to the Shango deity. A priest walks in, holding a prop chicken to offer in sacrifice. One man holds a knife, another a bowl in which to catch the (imagined) blood. After slitting the chicken's throat, the priest and the man with the bowl circle the stage, flicking blood on the participants. The participants sway and chant in response; the last one, the man with the knife, starts convulsing, his eyes rolling back in their sockets as he falls to the floor. He begins flicking his tongue, signaling that the Vodou loa Damballah has possessed him – an intercultural mixing of

Haiti and Trinidad that signaled Dunham taking creative liberties. He undulates his body like a snake, starting from pushing off his toes, rippling up through his legs, pelvis, spine, chest, neck, and head, to propel himself forward on the floor. The piece builds in energy as Shango takes over. In one section, a group of women bend their knees deeply, flexing at the waist to tilt their torsos forward over their knees, hands in fists at their chests with elbows out, and twist their spines (including their necks) side to side as they step to the beat in a right, left, right-left-right; left, right, left-right-left pattern, repeated to the point of exhaustion.[26]

Dances such as *Shango* inspired Black artists in France, Peru, Jamaica, Brazil, Canada, and elsewhere that the Dunham Company toured around the world from 1947 to 1960. Sometimes, these influences circled back to the very places she herself had drawn upon to develop her technique. One example is with Martinique. When Dunham visited in 1935, light-skinned, elite Martinicans – like elite Haitians – disavowed African cultural practices as "an unwanted symbol of a shameful past," instead enrolling their children in piano and ballet.[27] Dunham, free to ignore local class and race hierarchies, took inspiration from the Black working masses and their cultural practices, especially ladja, which she called *l'ag'ya*. Upon returning to the United States, she developed a 30-minute ballet, *L'Ag'Ya* (1938) that included a performance of ladja as well as other Martinican dances such as the beguine, mazouk, and majumba. *L'Ag'Ya* became a successful part of her touring repertory for the next 22 years. In 1948, Frantz Denis "Francisco" Charles, an elite Martinican living in Paris to pursue veterinary medicine, reached out to Dunham, whose company was currently performing there. Charles had taken ballet lessons as a child in Martinique and hoped to continue them in Europe. But upon seeing the Dunham Company perform, he abandoned veterinary medicine and ballet classes to become a Dunham dancer and drummer. After the Dunham company, he toured with the Fonseca African Ballet and then another troupe, *Los Africos*. In 1956 he returned to Martinique and shocked the community by performing in the capital city's Carnival parade with a *bèlè* drum. With Dunham's company, he had "lived

69

with black performers who valued their African ascendance" and no longer wanted to hide that side of him. He opened a nightclub, started a band, and became one of the largest influences on Martinican popular culture, reversing its centuries of the disavowal of Africanist cultural practices.[28]

In addition to her company's performances, Dunham's ethnographic writings and educational institutions also had widespread influence. As thousands of aspiring professional dancers flocked to the Dunham School in New York from 1944 to 1954, they absorbed new movement possibilities and disseminated them through their own choreography and teaching. One specific example of her influence in U.S. concert dance is the use of the pelvis. Many scholars have written about the multiple uses and meanings of pelvic movement in African diasporic dance forms.[29] Prior to Dunham, concert dance as developed in the 20th century in the United States had largely inherited Isadora Duncan's claim that American dance should have "no rhythm from the waist down."[30] Innovator Martha Graham did defy such a dictum and centered contractions of the pelvis into her dance technique, but a Graham contraction is unidirectional "concavity" in "the longitudinal body axis."[31] Dunham's technique and choreographic vocabulary, in contrast, demanded that a dancer move her pelvis polydirectionally and polyrhythmically. Contractions could undulate up the spine, as in the *yanvalou*, or initiate a full circle of the pelvis. A dancer could move his hips in a figure eight pattern, side to side in an undercurve, or in a semi-circular overcurve while stepping on the diagonal, as Talley Beatty does when approaching Dunham under an elevated train overpass in the film musical *Stormy Weather* (1943). Today, there is hardly a performance of modern, jazz, or contemporary dance that does not incorporate the more fluid, polyrhythmic, and varied use of the pelvis and spine that Dunham helped to disseminate.[32]

Dunham's influence also reached ballet. Brenda Dixon Gottschild has documented how famed choreographer George Balanchine was influenced by Africanist aesthetics through his working relationships with Josephine Baker, the Nicholas Brothers, and Dunham. What has often been called Balanchine's "neoclassical" or "American" style – speed, percussive attack, complex rhythmical patterning, flexed feet, increased mobility of the pelvis, and an over-all aesthetic of the cool – was, in fact, the influence of his Black collaborators.[33] Balanchine and Dunham worked together on the Black-cast Broadway musical *Cabin in the Sky* (1940). We can see her influence in the dance num-ber "(Vision) Egyptian Ballet," which immediately followed the song "My Old Virginia Home on the Nile." The lat-ter's title punned on the title of a popular minstrel song, "My Old Kentucky Home," written in 1853 by Stephen Foster, that invoked plantation nostalgia. With lyrics such as "The young folk roll/On the little cabin floor/All merry, all happy and bright," the song painted a picture of slave life as innocent and joyous.[34] Rather than reference a Southern plantation, Dunham's sequence imagines a different ances-tral home: Egypt. In the early 20th century, many Black Americans found inspiration in the powerful pharaohs, Black rulers who stood as proof of the greatness of African civilization. Langston Hughes' poem "The Negro Speaks of Rivers" (1921), in which the speaker "looked upon the Nile and built the pyramids above it," testifies to the alter-nate mythic past that ancient Egypt offered to people in the Diaspora.[35]

Balanchine wanted Dunham to wear a Bedouin costume and sing an Arabic tune, but she refused. His vision did not comport with the celebrated African past that she wanted to convey. Instead, her costume designer and husband John Pratt dressed her as Nefertiti, an Egyptian queen.[36] As we can see in Figure 3.1, Dunham's raised leg is turned out and bent in a balletic position (a front *attitude*), but she flexes her foot, which is bare. The carriage of her torso is erect and proud, but tilted and stylized. Drummers sit close to her, watching her movement. This arrangement was not just staged for a photograph. In the show, musicians did not sit in the orchestra pit, as was typical for Broadway perfor-mances, but performed onstage with her and her company, in close relationship, echoing Africanist aesthetic principles. Furthermore, she incorporated Caribbean movements into the choreography, drawing upon Haitian Vodou movements in particular for the "Hell" scene of the musical.

Whereas Balanchine's incorporation of these aesthetic elements would lead to celebrating him as the founder of neoclassical ballet, for Dunham they caused controversy. In their reviews of *Cabin*, theatre critics called her the "hottest thing on Broadway" and said that the company's dancing was "orgiastic."[37] Dunham tried to fight such perceptions in her article "Thesis Turned Broadway." In it, she argued that Caribbean dances could easily appear onstage in *Cabin in the Sky* if there were functional similarities. If the purpose of **the grouillère** in Haiti, for example, was to show "sexual stimulus and release" then it was acceptable to use the *grouillère* in *Cabin in the Sky*, when the functional context – sexual stimulation and release – was similar.[38] Dunham, however, failed to acknowledge that the broader context of these dances differed greatly. Working-class Haitians understood the dance as a part of commonplace social interaction, whereas middle-class American audiences attending a Broadway show read such movements as outside the boundary of normative sexuality.

The stickiness of translation raises the enduring doubleness of Black dance in the Americas – in the United States in particular. Hearkening back to W.E.B. DuBois' notion of "double consciousness," Thomas F. DeFrantz discusses the distinction between dances done for an in group, within a "circle that permits and protects," and dances that operate under a largely white gaze with a violent history. The white gaze echoes back to the slave ships crossing the Atlantic Ocean, where sailors forced enchained Africans to dance to keep up their physical fitness for the auction block.[39] The pleasure and power of Black social dance rub up against this history when performed for an audience. In the digital age, the lines between in-group witnessing and the external gaze can blur, as private meanings are often conveyed through the public-facing world of social media.

The case of hip hop dance is especially relevant here. Hip hop is a multifaceted cultural expression emerged from the boroughs of New York City, especially the South Bronx, during the 1970s. Original elements included emcee-ing (rapping), deejaying, visual art (graffiti), and breaking (dance). Practitioners speak of hip hop as a life-affirming ethos that challenges the social death ascribed to marginalized people, particularly people of African descent. Breaking embodies this philosophical aspect. Breaking battles typically take place in a circle, or cypher, in which individuals or groups of individuals compete in demonstrating corporeal intelligence with footwork, creative standing choreographies (uprocking), acrobatic spins and flips, derisive gestural "burns" of the opponent, and overall embodiment of the rhythm, which some call soul. Breaking crews assembled in the 1970s predominantly among young men. While hip hop overall is overwhelmingly identified with Black American culture, Puerto Rican dancers formed many of the second generation of breaking crews that became well known.[40]

In breaking, one can see the duality of Africanist aesthetics and the spirit of resistance to oppressive social conditions. Imani Kai Johnson calls the latter "outlaw culture," which "counters dominant notions about [South Bronx residents'] sociopolitical and racialized marginalization."[41] At the same time, Serouj Aprahamian cautions us not to characterize hip hop as a reactionary force. He writes, "the emancipatory power of the culture does not stem from it being a coping mechanism or reaction to negative stimuli...Rather, it lies in the culture itself."[42] Hip hop creatively reworked aesthetics honed by generations of working-class Black Americans, including connective threads of Africanist practices.

What happens when breaking goes global, and the two crews competing to win Battle of the Year in 2005 are from Japan and South Korea? In the documentary film *Planet B-Boy*, a member of Korea's Last for One crew shouts before they take the stage, "Dokdo Island is ours!"[43] Both South Korea and Japan claim sovereignty over this territory (known in English as the Liancourt Rocks), a dispute that dates back over 300 years but is more recently linked to Japan's oppressive imperial rule over Korea from 1905 to 1945.[44] The burns and acrobatic one-upmanship of 2005's Final Battle of the Year operated in a context of friction

between two Asian nations. From one perspective, this contextual translation is an example of what DeFrantz calls hip
hop's "performative flexibility"; from the other, it divorces
breaking from the specific struggles of people of African
descent in the Americas.[45] Imani Kai Johnson notes that in
conversations at competitions, breakers articulate stereotypes
that Asian dancers are too technical and soulless, echoing
jingoistic "**Yellow Peril**" discourses that see Asian nations
as a threat to U.S. power. Several of these Asian dancers,
however, *live* hip hop; the dance has "claimed" them, and
the stereotypes of soullessness float free of how they actually move on the competition stage and in their everyday
lives. Given that breaking is now central to South Korean
national culture, with the "full endorsement" of the government, Johnson questions whether Korea may become a part
of the history that breakers should know. At the same time,
the "soulfulness" attributed to breaking, a way-of-being-in-
the-world that goes beyond the steps, remains rooted in its
connections to the African diaspora.[46]

What Kariamu Welsh Asante called "epic memory" and
Esailama Diouf "spirit talk" endures in writings about
African diasporic dance as a mode of connecting to divin-
ity and ancestry simultaneously.[47] Depending on the writer's
positionality and approach, however, such a broad characterization can sound not only essentialist – meaning, defining
a group of people by qualities falsely perceived to be natural or "essential" – but also exoticizing, a dance version of
the "magical Negro" trope of Hollywood film and television that attributes extra capacity for soulfulness to people
of African descent while ignoring the violent repercussions
of superhumanization.[48] Jasmine Johnson reminds us that
from the Middle Passage onward, Black dance has had a
"continued relationship to the project of white supremacy:
coerced movement to satiate white appetites for capital
and control."[49] It is this ambivalence that Black dancers in
the United States in particular continue to face. TikTok,
a social media outlet for sharing innovative expressions
quickly turned into a vehicle for white appropriation, to the
point where Black TikTok creators declared a strike in the
summer of 2021.[50] While keeping in mind such potential

landmines when speaking broadly, the life-affirming ethos of dances in the African diaspora continues to draw people to them. The shout of *Ase!*, a Yoruban term that speaks to such a powerful life force, can be heard in a capoeira *roda* in Brazil or in a Dunham Technique class in the United States. Imani Johnson speaks of feeling that ineffable sense of collective unity in breaking cyphers across the world.[51] Dance in the African diaspora expands capaciously, with definitions of Africanist, diasporic, or Black in constant negotiation.

## FURTHER READING

Daniel, Yvonne. *Dancing Wisdom: Embodied Knowledge in Haitian Vodou, Cuban Yoruba, and Bahian Candomblé*. Urbana: University of Illinois, 2005. *Dancing Wisdom* argues that dance is a central component of African diasporic religious practices in the circum-Caribbean. She analyzes the aesthetic and philosophical components of Vodou, Yoruba, and Candomblé through ethnographic fieldwork and combines that with theoretical work on African diasporic religions. By investigating three different forms, she showcases distinctions as well as similarities.

DeFrantz, Thomas F. and Anita Gonzalez, eds. *Black Performance Theory*. Durham, NC: Duke University Press, 2014. This book assembles many of the most important scholars of Black Dance, Theatre, and Performance Studies. The authors tackle globalization, the digital information revolution, new expressions of gender and sexuality, challenges to essentialized identity categories, and the turn to diaspora as a "meta-discourse" in their analyses of Black performance. DeFrantz and Gonzalez's introduction, which provides a genealogy of how generations of scholars have addressed questions about Blackness in relation to performance, is particularly useful.

Gottschild, Brenda Dixon. *Digging the Africanist Presence in American Performance: Dance and Other Contexts*. Westport: Greenwood Press, 1996. Dr Gottschild's book transformed dance studies by challenging the perceived whiteness of concert dance genres such as ballet, modern, and postmodern dance. Terms that she coins in this book, such as "invisibilization" and "Africanist," have become standard in analyzing how dance operates in the United States.

Welsh, Kariamu, Esailama G.A. Diouf, and Yvonne Daniel, eds. *Hot Feet and Social Change: African Dance and Diaspora Communities*.

Urbana: University of Illinois Press, 2019. This recent book, edited by some of the most important scholars in African diasporic dance studies, showcases the breadth and richness of African dance in the Americas, particularly the United States. Far from viewing African influence as something of the pre-modern past, these authors demonstrate how West, Central, and South African dancers, musicians, and choreographers have influenced dance in the United States in the 20th and 21st centuries.

# TIMELINE

1525 – Middle Passage begins. For the next 300-plus years, Portuguese, Dutch, British, French, Spanish, and other European nations enslave Africans and transport them to the Western Hemisphere.

16th–19th century – Enslaved Africans in the Western Hemisphere continue dance traditions from their homelands and develop new ones. Religious practices that incorporate dance include Vodou in Haiti, Santería in Cuba, Candomblé in Brazil, Hoodoo in Louisiana, and Obeah throughout the Caribbean. Martial art dance forms, such as capoeira in Brazil and ladja/danmyé in Martinique, also develop, as well as countless social dances, such as the Cakewalk in the Southern United States and tango in Argentina.

1840s – William Henry Lane, or "Master Juba," showcases his innovative blend of West African aesthetics and Irish jigging to become one of the most famous stage performers in the world. Countless white men in blackface imitate him in the new theatrical genre of minstrelsy, which develops in the United States. Lane's dance aesthetics become influential in the development of tap, jazz, and step dancing.

1860s–1880s – Black US Americans replace white performers in minstrel shows, further innovating and refining Black social dances for the theatrical stage.

1890s–1910s – In the United States, Aida Overton Walker and other Black US American choreographers transition from minstrelsy to vaudeville, shedding blackface and caricatured stereotypes to promote revised performances of the Cakewalk and other ragtime dances.

1920s – The international New Negro Movement promotes the celebration of African cultural roots and asserts a new political consciousness in challenging white supremacy, colonialism, and imperialism. Martinican Aimé Cesaire coins the term *negritude*, roughly understood as a Black consciousness. In Cuba, there is the Afro-Cubanismo movement; in Haiti, the indigenisme movement; in the United

States, the Harlem Renaissance. Africanist dance aesthetics become central to stage performances across the Americas. On Broadway, tap and jazz dominate.

1930s – Katherine Dunham and Zora Neale Hurston, Black US Americans, conduct ethnographic research in the Caribbean and document many dance forms, including the shay-shay in Jamaica, the mazouk in Martinique, and the beguine in Haiti. Dunham begins to incorporate these dances into her choreography, performed on Broadway and on stages across the globe.1940s–1960s – Across the Americas, national dance troupes are formed that highlight and promote Africanist aesthetics, including the National Dance Theatre Company of Jamaica, founded by Rex Nettleford. Individuals such as Jean-Leon Destiné of Haiti and Alvin Ailey in the United States form their own companies, not necessarily tied to a national identity, and tour the world. Afro-Caribbean social dances such as mambo, rhumba, and calypso become the rage across the Americas.

1960s – The Black Arts Movement emerges in the United States, which reaffirms the social and political consciousness of Black art and the need to turn to Africa, instead of Europe, for aesthetic principles and practices. West African music and dance classes become a part of dance studios, community centers, and higher education curricula.

1970s–1980s – In New York City, breaking emerges as a popular dance form. On the West Coast, popping, locking, and whaacking develop. By the 1980s, these aesthetics merge to become known as hip hop dance. Breaking is featured in the 1984 Summer Olympics Opening Ceremony in Los Angeles.

1980s–2000s – Hip hop, Michael Jackson's choreography, and other Africanist-based dance forms spread across the globe, aided by MTV and other means of dissemination.

2000s–2020s – Greater acknowledgment of the Africanist roots of dance innovations in the Americas across all sectors of dance – concert dance, Broadway dance, popular entertainment, and social dance. Debates about cultural appropriation and the stealing of Black dances increase with the proliferation of social media platforms such as YouTube and TikTok that make such dances go "viral."

# REFERENCES

Amin, Takiyah Nur. "A Terminology of Difference: Making the Case for Black Dance in the 21st Century and Beyond." In *Journal of Pan African Studies* vol. 4, no. 6 (September 2011):7–15.

Aprahamian, Serouj. "Hip-Hop, Gangs, and the Criminalization of African American Culture: A Critical Aprpaisal of *Yes Yes Y'all*." *Journal of Black Studies* 50, no. 3 (2019): 298–315.

Asante, Kariamu Welsh. "Commonalities in African Dance: An Aesthetic Foundation." In *African Culture: The Rhythms of Unity*, 71–82. Edited by Molefi Kete Asante and Kariamu Welsh Asante. Westport: Greenwood Press, 1985.

Bambara, Celia Weiss. "Yanvalou's Elliptic Displacements: Staging Spirit Time in the United States." *Journal of Haitian Studies* 15, no. 1–2 (2009): 290–303.

Bannerman, Henrietta. "An Overview of the Development of Martha Graham's Movement System." *Dance Research: The Journal of the Society for Dance Research* 17, no. 2 (1999): 9–46.

Césaire, Aimé. *The Original 1939 Notebook of a Return to the Native Land*. Edited and translated by A. James Arnold and Layton Eshleman. Middletown, CT: Wesleyan University Press, 2013 [1939].

Corbett, Saroya. "Katherine Dunham's Mark on Jazz Dance." In *Jazz Dance: A History of the Roots and Branches*, edited by Lindsay Guarino and Wendy Oliver, 89–96. Gainesville: University Press of Florida, 2014.

Cyrille, Dominique. "Popular Music and Martinican-Creole Identity." *Black Music Research Journal* 22, no. 1 (2002): 65–83.

Das, Joanna Dee. "Dancing Dahomey at the World's Fair: Revising the Archive of African Dance." In *Futures of Dance Studies*, 56–73. Edited by Susan Manning, Janice Ross, and Rebecca Schneider. Madison: University of Wisconsin Press, 2019.

Dash, Michael J. *The Other America: Caribbean Literature in a New World Context*. Charlottesville: University Press of Virginia, 1998.

DeFrantz, Thomas F. "The Black Beat Made Visible: Hip Hop Dance and Body Power." In *Of the Presence of the Body: Essays on Dance and Performance Theory*, edited by André Lepecki, 64–81, Middletown, CT: Wesleyan University Press, 2004.

DeFrantz, Thomas F. "Foreword: Black Bodies Dancing Black Culture—Black Atlantic Transformations." In *EmBODYing Liberation: The Black Body in American Dance*, edited by Dorothea Fischer-Hornung and Alison D. Goeller, 11–16. Hamburg, Germany: LIT, 2001.

DeFrantz, Thomas F. "Hip Hop Habitus 2.0." In *Black Performance Theory*, edited by Thomas F. DeFrantz and Anita Gonzalez. Durham, NC: Duke University Press, 2014.

DeFrantz, Thomas F. "What is Black Dance? What Can It Do?" In *Thinking Through Theatre and Performance*, edited by Maaike Bleeker, Adrian Kear, Joe Kelleher, and Heike Roms, 87–99. London: Methuen Drama, 2019.

DeFrantz, Thomas F. and Anita Gonzalez, eds. *Black Performance Theory*. Durham, NC: Duke University Press, 2014.

Duncan, Isadora. "I See America Dancing." Orig. pub. 1927. In Isadora Duncan, *The Art of the Dance*, edited by Sheldon Cheney. New York: Theatre Arts Books, 1977.

Dunham, Katherine. "Form and Function in Primitive Dance." *Educational Dance* 4, no. 1 (1941).

Dunham, Katherine. "Thesis Turned Broadway." Orig. pub. 1941. In *Kaiso! Writings by and about Katherine Dunham*, edited by Vévé Clark and Sara E. Johnson, 214-216. Madison: University of Wisconsin Press, 2005.

Edwards, Brent Hayes. *The Practice of Diaspora: Literature, Translation, and the Rise of Black Internationalism*. Cambridge: Harvard University Press, 2003.

Emery, Lynn. *Black Dance from 1619–Today*. Second Edition. Princeton, NJ: Princeton Book Company, 1989.

Fleurant, Gerdès. *Dancing Spirits: Rhythms and Rituals of Haitian Vodun, the Rada Rite*. Westport, CT: Greenwood Press, 1996.

Geggus, David. "The Bois Caïman Ceremony." *Journal of Caribbean History* 25, no. 1 (1991): 41–57.

Gottschild, Brenda Dixon. *Digging the Africanist Presence in American Performance: Dance and Other Contexts*. Westport: Greenwood Press, 1996.

Gilroy, Paul. *The Black Atlantic: Modernity and Double-Consciousness*. Cambridge: Harvard University Press, 1993.

Hall, Stuart. "Cultural Identity and Diaspora." In *Identity: Community, Culture, Difference*, 222–237. Edited by Jonathan Rutherford. London: Lawrence & Wishart, 1990.

Hazzard-Donald, Katrina. "Dance in Hip Hop Culture." In *Droppin' Science: Critical Essays on Rap Music and Hip Hop Culture*, edited by William Eric Perkins, 220–235. Philadelphia: Temple University Press, 1996.

Herskovits, Melville Jean. *The Myth of the Negro Past*. New York: Harper & Brothers, 1941.

Höfling, Ana Paula. *Staging Brazil: Choreographies of Capoeira*. Middletown: Wesleyan University Press, 2019.

Johnson, Imani Kai. "Battling in the Bronx: Social Choreography and Outlaw Culture Among Early Hip-Hop Streetdancers in New York City." *Dance Research Journal* 50, no. 2 (2018): 62–75.

Johnson, Imani Kai. "Black Culture Without Black People: Hip Hop Dance Beyond Appropriation Discourse." In *Are You Entertained?: Black Popular Culture in the Twenty-First Century*, edited by Simone C. Drake and Dwan K. Henderson, 191–206. Durham: Duke University Press, 2020.

Johnson, Imani Kai. "B-Boying and Battling in a Global Context: The Discursive Life of Difference in Hip Hop Dance." *Alif* 31 (2011): 173–195.

Johnson, Jasmine. "Black Laws of Dance." *Conversations Across the Field of Dance Studies: Decolonizing Dance Discourses.* Dance Studies Association, XL (2020): 25–27.

LaMothe, Mario. "*Dedouble* and Jeanguy Saintus' Corporeal Gifts." *E-Misférica* 12, no. 1 (2015), https://hemi.nyu.edu/hemi/pt/emisferica-121-caribbean-rasanblaj/lamothe.

Moore, Robin. *Nationalizing Blackness: Afrocubanismo and Artistic Revolution in Havana, 1920–1940.* Pittsburgh, PA: University of Pittsburgh Press, 1997.

Pan, Lu. *Aestheticizing Public Space: Street Visual Politics in East Asian Cities.* Bristol, UK: Intellect, 2015.

Polyné, Millery. "'To Carry the Dance of the People Beyond': Jean León Destiné, Lavinia Williams, and *Danse Folklorique Haitienne.*" *Journal of Haitian Studies* 10 (2004): 33–51.

Ramsey, Kate. *The Spirits and the Law: Vodou and Power in Haiti.* Chicago: University of Chicago Press, 2011.

Ramsey, Kate. "Vodou, Nationalism, and Performance: The Staging of Folklore in Mid-Twentieth-Century Haiti." In *Meaning in Motion: New Cultural Studies of Dance,* edited by Jane Desmond, 345–378. Durham, NC: Duke University Press, 1997.

Schloss, Joseph. *Foundation: B-boys, B-girls and Hip-Hop Culture in New York.* New York: Oxford, 2009.

Schomburg, Arthur. "The Negro Digs up His Past." In *The New Negro,* edited by Alain Locke. New York: A. & C. Boni, 1925.

Stearns, Jean and Marshall. *Jazz Dance: The Story of American Vernacular Dance.* New York: Da Capo Press, 1994.

Thompson, Robert Farris. "An Aesthetic of the Cool: West African Dance." In *African Forum* vol. 2, no. 2 (Fall 1966): 85–102.

Thompson, Robert Farris. *Tango: The Art History of Love.* New York: Vintage, 2006.

Waytz, Adam, Kelly Marie Hoffman, and Sophie Trawalter. "A Superhumanization Bias in Whites' Perceptions of Blacks." *Social Psychological and Personality Science,* Oct 8, 2014, DOI: 10.1177/1948550614553642.

Welsh, Kariamu, Esailama G.A. Diouf, and Yvonne Daniel, eds. *Hot Feet and Social Change: African Dance and Diaspora Communities.* Urbana: University of Illinois Press, 2019.

Wilson, Carlton. "Conceptualizing the African Diaspora." *Comparative Studies of South Asia, Africa and the Middle East* 17, no. 2 (1997): 118–122.

# NOTES

1  "Ag'ya, Martinique Fieldwork, 1936," Filmed by Katherine Dunham, Video Clip #18, Library of Congress, www.loc. gov/item/ihas.200003825/0:53-1:10.

2  The first time I introduce a term in a non-English language, I will italicize it, but not thereafter.

3  Kariamu Welsh, Esailama G.A. Diouf, and Yvonne Daniel, *Hot Feet and Social Change: African Dance and Diaspora Communities* (Urbana: University of Illinois Press, 2019), 1.

4  Carlton Wilson, "Conceptualizing the African Diaspora," *Comparative Studies of South Asia, Africa and the Middle East* 17, no. 2 (1997): 118; Stuart Hall, "Cultural Identity and Diaspora," in *Identity: Community, Culture, Difference*, ed. Jonathan Rutherford (London: Lawrence & Wishart, 1990); Paul Gilroy, *The Black Atlantic: Modernity and Double-Consciousness* (Cambridge: Harvard University Press, 1993); Brent Hayes Edwards, *The Practice of Diaspora: Literature, Translation, and the Rise of Black Internationalism* (Cambridge: Harvard University Press, 2003).

5  Brenda Dixon Gottschild, *Digging the Africanist Presence in American Performance: Dance and Other Contexts* (Westport: Greenwood Press, 1996), xiv. For more on the Africanist influence on ballet and tango, see Gottschild, *Digging the Africanist Presence in American Performance*, 59–80; Robert Farris Thompson, *Tango: The Art History of Love* (New York: Vintage, 2006).

6  Robert Farris Thompson, "An Aesthetic of the Cool: West African Dance," *African Forum* 2, no. 2 (Fall 1966): 85–102.

7  Jean and Marshall Stearns, *Jazz Dance: The Story of American Vernacular Dance* (New York: Da Capo Press, 1994 [1968]), 15.

8  Kariamu Welsh Asante, "Commonalities in African Dance: An Aesthetic Foundation," in *African Culture: The Rhythms of Unity*, ed. Molefi Kete Asante and Kariamu Welsh Asante, 71–82 (Westport: Greenwood Press, 1985).

9  Gottschild, *Digging the Africanist Presence in American Performance*, 11–19.

10  Ana Paula Höfling, *Staging Brazil: Choreographies of Capoeira* (Middletown: Wesleyan University Press, 2019), 11–13; Joanna Dee Das, "Dancing Dahomey at the World's Fair: Revising the Archive of African Dance," in *Futures of Dance Studies*, ed. Susan Manning, Janice Ross, and Rebecca Schneider (Madison: University of Wisconsin Press, 2020), 56–73; Welsh, Diouf, and Daniel, *Hot Feet and Social Change*.

11  Nadine George-Graves, "Diasporic Spidering: Constructing Contemporary Black Identities," in *Black Performance Theory*, ed. Thomas F. DeFrantz and Anita Gonzalez (Durham, NC: Duke University Press, 2014), 43.

12 Thomas F. DeFrantz and Anita Gonzalez, "Introduction: From 'Negro Expression' to 'Black Performance,'" *Black Performance Theory*, 5–6.

13 Takiyah Nur Amin, "Making the Case for Black Dance," *Journal of Pan African Studies* 4, no. 6 (2011): 7–15.

14 Thomas F. DeFrantz, "What is Black Dance? What Can It Do?" in *Thinking Through Theatre and Performance*, ed. Maaike Bleeker, Adrian Kear, Joe Kelleher, and Heike Roms (London: Methuen Drama, 2019), 87–89.

15 Aimé Césaire, *The Original 1939 Notebook of a Return to the Native Land*, ed. and trans. A. James Arnold and Layton Eshleman (Middletown, CT: Wesleyan University Press, 2013 [1939]), 19. This translation states, "where negritude rose for the first time," but most texts use the "stood up" translation. See Michael J. Dash, *The Other America: Caribbean Literature in a New World Context* (Charlottesville: University Press of Virginia, 1998), 62. For more on Vodou, see Margarite Fernández Olmos and Lizabeth Paravisini-Gebert, *Creole Religions of the Caribbean: An Introduction from Vodou and Santería to Obeah and Espiritismo* (New York: New York University Press, 2003); David Geggus offers doubt about the ceremony. See "The Bois Caïman Ceremony," *Journal of Caribbean History*, 41–57. Nonetheless, Kate Ramsey avers that "magico-religious beliefs served to mobilize resistance and foster a revolutionary mentality." See Kate Ramsey, *The Spirits and the Law: Vodou and Power in Haiti* (Chicago: University of Chicago Press, 2011), 42–44.

16 Celia Weiss Bambara, "Yanvalou's Elliptic Displacements: Staging Spirit Time in the United States," *Journal of Haitian Studies* 15, no. 1–2 (2009): 293.

17 Gerdès Fleurant, *Dancing Spirits: Rhythms and Rituals of Haitian Vodun, the Rada Rite* (Westport, CT: Greenwood Press, 1996), 25; Katherine Dunham, "Thesis Turned Broadway," orig. pub. 1941, in *Kaiso! Writings by and about Katherine Dunham*, ed. VéVé Clark and Sara E. Johnson, 214–216 (Madison: University of Wisconsin Press, 2005); Katherine Dunham, "Form and Function in Primitive Dance," *Educational Dance* 4, no. 1 (1941): 3.

18 Melville Jean Herskovits, *The Myth of the Negro Past* (New York: Harper & Brothers, 1941), 1.

19 Kate Ramsey, *The Spirits and the Law*, 177.

20 Jean Price-Mars, *So Spoke the Uncle [Ainsi parla l'oncle]*, trans. Magdaline W. Shannon (Washington, DC: Three Continents Press, 1983 [1928]).

21 See Arthur Schomburg, "The Negro Digs up His Past," in *The New Negro: An Interpretation*, ed. Alain Locke, 231–237 (New York: A. & C. Boni, 1925); Robin Moore, *Nationalizing Blackness: Afrocubanismo and Artistic Revolution in Havana, 1920–1940* (Pittsburgh, PA: University of Pittsburgh Press, 1997).

22  For more, see Millery Polyné, "'To carry the dance of the people beyond': Jean Leon Destiné, Lavinia Williams, and Danse Folklorique Haitienne." *Journal of Haitian Studies* 10 (2004): 33–51; Kate Ramsey, "Vodou, Nationalism, and Performance: The Staging of Folklore in Mid-Twentieth-Century Haiti," in *Meaning in Motion: New Cultural Studies of Dance*, ed. Jane Desmond, 345–378 (Durham, NC: Duke University Press, 1997).

23  Jeanguy Saintus, quoted in Catherine Annie Hollingsworth, "Jeanguy Saintus: Contretemps," *The Miami Rail*, September 28, 2016, https://miamirail.org/performing-arts/jeanguy-saintus-contretemps/.

24  Mario LaMothe, "*Dedouble* and Jeanguy Saintus' Corporeal Gifts," *E-Misférica* 12, no. 1 (2015), https://hemi.nyu.edu/hemi/pt/emisferica-121-caribbean-rasanblaj/lamothe; "Jeanguy Saintus on a New *Rite of Spring*," Opera North, February 11, 2019, www.operanorth.co.uk/news/jeanguy-saintus-on-a-new-rite-of-spring/.

25  E. Lescot, "In Appreciation," *Tropics and Le Jazz "Hot"* Program, April 28, 1940, Jerome Robbins Dance Division; Kate Ramsey, "Katherine Dunham and the Folklore Performance Movement in Post-US Occupation Haiti," in Chin, *Katherine Dunham*, 65–66.

26  Katherine Dunham, "Shango," filmed 1947 by Ann Barzel at the Studebaker Theater in Chicago, Library of Congress, www.loc.gov/item/ihas.200003834/.; *The Magic of Katherine Dunham*, dress rehearsal, Alvin Ailey American Dance Theater, 1987, VHS, Jerome Robbins Dance Division, New York Public Library for the Performing Arts.

27  Dominique Cyrille, "Popular Music and Martinican-Creole Identity," *Black Music Research Journal* 22, no. 1 (2002): 69.

28  Cyrille, "Popular Music and Martinican-Creole Identity," 71–72.

29  Adanna Kai Jones, Melissa Blanco-Borelli.

30  Isadora Duncan, "I See America Dancing," orig. pub. 1927, in Isadora Duncan, *The Art of the Dance*, ed. Sheldon Cheney (New York: Theatre Arts Books, 1977), 48.

31  Billie Lepcyzk, quoted in Henrietta Bannerman, "An Overview of the Development of Martha Graham's Movement System," *Dance Research: The Journal of the Society for Dance Research* 17, no. 2 (1999): 37.

32  *Stormy Weather*, directed by Andrew Stone, (1943, Los Angeles: 20th Century Fox, 2006), DVD. For more on Katherine Dunham's influence, see Joanna Dee Das, *Katherine Dunham: Dance and the African Diaspora* (New York: Oxford, 2017), and Saroya Corbett, "Katherine Dunham's Mark on Jazz Dance," in *Jazz Dance: A History of the Roots and Branches*, ed. Lindsay Guarino and Wendy Oliver, 89–96 (Gainesville: University Press of Florida, 2014).

33 See Gottschild, *Digging the Africanist Presence in American Performance*, 59–79.

34 Arthur Knight, *Disintegrating the Musical: Black Performance and American Musical Film* (Durham: Duke University Press, 2002), 126–127; Richard Jackson, *Stephen Foster's Songbook: Original Sheet Music of 40 Songs by Stephen Collins Foster* (Mineola, NY: Dover Musical Archives, 1974).

35 Iris Schmeisser, "'Ethiopia shall soon stretch forth her hands': Ethiopianism, Egyptomania, and the Arts of the Harlem Renaissance," in *African Diasporas in the New and Old Worlds: Consciousness and Imagination*, ed. Genevieve Fabre and Klaus Benesch (Amsterdam: Rodopi, 2004), 265–266; Langston Hughes, "The Negro Speaks of Rivers," AAC audio file, *The Voice of Langston Hughes*, Smithsonian Folkways Recordings, 1995, www.folkways.si.edu/TrackDetails.aspx?itemid=32941.

36 Dunham, interview by Hill, January 15, 2000.

37 "Hottest Thing on Broadway," *Sunday News*, December 8, 1940, Box 2, Series 3, Folder 2, J. Rosamond Johnson Papers, Yale University; "'Cabin in the Sky' Sepia Fantasy of Heaven—Earth—and Hell," *New York City Retailing*, November 4, 1940, Katherine Dunham Papers, Southern Illinois University, Box 102, Folder 6; "Katherine Dunham and Ethel Waters Continue To Steal The Spotlight," *Philadelphia Independent*, November 17, 1940, Box 102, Folder 6, Katherine Dunham Papers, Southern Illinois University.

38 Katherine Dunham, "Thesis Turned Broadway," orig. pub. 1941, reprinted in *Kaiso! Writings by and About Katherine Dunham*, ed. VéVé Clark and Sara E. Johnson, 214–216 (Madison: University of Wisconsin Press, 2005). Dunham further discusses "sexual stimulation and release" in "Form and Function in Primitive Dance," *Educational Dance* 4, no. 1 (1941): 2–4.

39 DeFrantz, "Foreword: Black Bodies Dancing Black Culture—Black Atlantic Transformations," in *EmBODYing Liberation: The Black Body in American Dance*, edited by Dorothea Fischer-Hornung and Alison D. Goeller, 11 (Hamburg, Germany: LIT, 2001); Thomas F. DeFrantz, "The Black Beat Made Visible: Hip Hop Dance and Body Power," in *Of the Presence of the Body: Essays on Dance and Performance Theory*, edited by André Lepecki (Middletown, CT: Wesleyan University Press, 2004), 64; Lynn Emery, *Black Dance from 1619–Today*, Second Edition (Princeton, NJ: Princeton Book Company, 1989), 6.

40 For more on the history of hip hop dance, see Katrina Hazzard-Donald, "Dance in Hip Hop Culture," in *Droppin' Science: Critical Essays on Rap Music and Hip Hop Culture*, ed. William Eric Perkins, 220–235 (Philadelphia: Temple University Press, 1996); Joseph Schloss, *Foundation: B-boys, B-girls and Hip-Hop Culture in New York* (New York: Oxford, 2009).

41  Imani Kai Johnson, "Battling in the Bronx: Social Choreography and Outlaw Culture Among Early Hip-Hop Streetdancers in New York City," *Dance Research Journal* 50, no. 2 (2018): 63.

42  Serouj Aprahamian, "Hip-Hop, Gangs, and the Criminalization of African American Culture: A Critical Appraisal of *Yes Yes Y'all*," *Journal of Black Studies* 50, no. 3 (2019): 311.

43  Benson Lee, *Planet B-Boy*, Elephant Eye Films, USA, 2008.

44  Alexandra Genova, "Two Nations Disputed These Islands for 300 Years," *National Geographic*, November 14, 2018, accessed November 29, 2021, www.nationalgeographic.com/travel/article/history-dispute-photos-dodko-rocks-islands.

45  Thomas F. DeFrantz, "Hip Hop Habitus 2.0," in *Black Performance Theory*, 231.

46  Imani Kai Johnson, "B-Boying and Battling in a Global Context: The Discursive Life of Difference in Hip Hop Dance," *Alif* 31 (2011): 182, 190. For more on breaking in South Korea, see Lu Pan, *Aestheticizing Public Space: Street Visual Politics in East Asian Cities* (Bristol, UK: Intellect, 2015), 24–26; Victoria Namkung, "Seoul's Bumping B-Boy Scene," *New York Times*, December 16, 2017, www.nytimes.com/2017/12/16/style/south-korea-hip-hop-breakdancing-seoul.html; for more on dance claiming people, see Johnson, "Black Culture Without Black People: Hip Hop Dance Beyond Appropriation Discourse," in *Are You Entertained?: Black Popular Culture in the Twenty-First Century*, ed. Simone C. Drake and Dwan K. Henderson, 191–206 (Durham: Duke University Press, 2020).

47  Esailama G.A. Diouf, "Sauce! Conjuring the African Dream in America through Dance," in *Hot Feet and Social Change*, 20–27.

48  Adam Waytz, Kelly Marie Hoffman, and Sophie Trawalter, "A Superhumanization Bias in Whites' Perceptions of Blacks," *Social Psychological and Personality Science*, Oct 8, 2014, DOI: 10.1177/1948550614553642.

49  Jasmine Johnson, "Black Laws of Dance," *Conversations Across the Field of Dance Studies: Decolonizing Dance Discourses*, Dance Studies Association, XL (2020): 26.

50  Sharon Pruitt-Young, "Black TikTok Creators Are On Strike To Protest A Lack of Credit For Their Work," NPR, July 1, 2021, www.npr.org/2021/07/01/1011899328/black-tiktok-creators-are-on-strike-to-protest-a-lack-of-credit-for-their-work.

51  Imani Johnson, presentation to Washington University Performing Arts Department Colloquium, December 4, 2020, Zoom.

# CHAPTER 4

# Ballet

## From Louis XIV to Misty Copeland

*Sekani Robinson*

In the seventh grade, I had a dream about a Black ballerina. In my dream, I couldn't see the ballerina's face, but she had dark skin and curly hair like mine. This dream led me to write a poem about this mysterious dancer, for an English class assignment. The poem started with, "This beautiful Black dancer dances to hide her tears. She dances to hide her fears. She dances to forget her anger and sorrow… I don't know who this Black dancer is but she's dancing to help make the community grow." After writing the poem, I realized that despite having studied ballet since I was three years old, I had never actually seen a ballerina on stage that looked like me, and so I began a journey to find her.

I searched online and came across an article with a picture of Aesha Ash – a graceful and elegant Black ballet dancer wearing a beautiful orange costume. The title of the article was "Where Are All the Black Swans?" by Gia Koulas for *The New York Times*. It criticized major ballet companies for their lack of diversity and specifically, their lack of Black women in ballet. My dream, my poem, and this article sent me on a dance history voyage. Thirteen years later, I am still filling in the gaps of where all of the Black dancers reside within the canon of dance history. Black dancers and creatives have contributed to many aspects of the artform. This chapter traces my investigation of the history of classical, neoclassical, and contemporary ballet as it pertains to the conflict of diversity and elitism in the world of ballet.

DOI: 10.4324/9781003185918-4

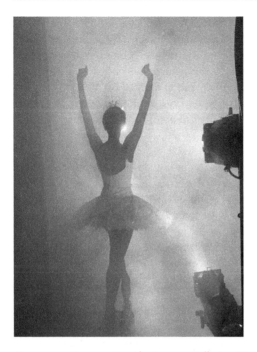

**Figure 4.1:** Dancer: Paunika Jones – Ballerina/Yogi and Budding Artistic Director, IG: paunikaj. Photographer: Leonard Perez – Dances with Collage Dance Collective: IG: leonardperezjr. Title: "Everything about my entire existence is a protest"

Since its inception in Italy during the late 14th and early 15th centuries, ballet has been an activity enjoyed and practiced by predominantly white Europeans. Originally ballet was strictly for royal courtiers. The origins of the term ballet originate from the Italian word *ballare*. During this time, ballet resembled a cotillion or debutant style social dance. Its purpose was to display social etiquette which typically is performed at/for a formal ball. Being so, the royal courts employed dance experts who trained aristocrats in dance and music, so that they could perform at dance halls with other aristocrats.

In 1533, Catherine de Medici, a young noble from Florence, Italy, married the soon-to-be French King Henry II and moved to France. She brought with her architects, woodworkers, artisans, and perhaps most importantly *ballet de cour* or ballet of the court. Medici introduced early styles of dance to court life in France. This began the expansion of ballet amongst the royals in France. By the 17th century, approximately 100 years later, under the reign of French King Louis XIV, ballet had transformed into the artform we experience today.

King Louis XIV was so intrigued by ballet that he himself became a talented dancer. He would be nicknamed "the Dancing King" and in 1661, he formed the Académie Royale de Danse right next to his grand home – the Palace of Versailles. The Académie Royale de Danse became the first state-funded school for ballet. The school shifted from court dance to a **proscenium** form and codified the technique of what is now considered classical ballet.[1]

Dance scholar Maureen Needham states,

> The Académie Royale de Danse did indeed function as a true academy, where thirteen experts met regularly to deliberate on ways to improve artistic standards.... [They also had to] pass aesthetic judgment upon every newly choreographed dance, both social and theatrical, before it could be either taught or performed in Paris.[2]

This created state censorship within the ballet form which played a major role in King Louis's ability to dominate his nobles both socially and politically. He knew how to use dance to control his court, keeping his enemies close and satiated through parties and fêtes that ensured his reign. It also created an exclusivity of what can be done within ballet and who has access to the artform. This ideology has evolved in various ways but nevertheless, still impacts cultural equity in the field today.

The 17th century is the Baroque Ballet era, the golden age of French classical art and culture. French aesthetics would expand across Europe and in 1689, ballet reached Moscow. In Russia, as in France, ballet was used as a way to maintain authority over its people. Ballet in Russia represented a form of physical conformity of idealism for its creators and the masses. Ballet became the embodiment of Russian imperialism.[3]

During the 17th and 18th centuries, ballet in Russia flourished, resulting in the creation of the Mariinsky Ballet in 1738 by Empress Anna Ioannovna. She had appointed renowned French dancer Jean-Baptiste Landé seven years earlier to establish the Imperial Theatre School in St. Petersburg's Palace where he trained young dancers in classical ballet.[4] He not only assisted in building Russian ballet, but he also influenced the long-held traditions of French ballet. Classical ballet schools and companies flourished in Russia and soon extended outside of the royal courts. In 1776 the Bolshoi Ballet was founded with the intent to provide Moscow orphans the opportunity to achieve stardom through their ballet training. However, the Bolshoi struggled to compete with Landé's Mariinsky Ballet, and it was not until the 1900s when renowned choreographer Alexander Gorsky was appointed ballet master of Bolshoi Ballet that its own style developed.

Following the French Revolution (1789–1799) and the fall of the aristocracy, the Romantic era ballets would embody the socio-political shifts of the early 1800s. The Romantic era was a backlash to the French aristocracy. This was a time of artistic reaction against the formality and strict regulations of neoclassicism. Society was divided into nobles and clergy on one side and the working class on the other. Nobles were no longer revered characters in ballets, as they fell from grace. Instead, morality stories that focused on the lives of the middle class would ascend. The romantic ballets included three repeating themes: nobles who made bad love choices, unrequited love resulting in death, and gravity-defying unearthly creatures whose roles accentuated an advancing pointe work. The shift to Romanticism affected gender roles as well. Until the 1820s, the roles of men and women were on par with one another; but as ballet themes transitioned, men were minimized to support the ballerina through the tasks of lifting and supporting the ballerina in various attitudes, turns, and sporadic leaps.[5] These parallels are captured in the iconic ballets *La Sylphide* (1832) and *Giselle* (1841) which both premiered in Paris during this time.

Also, during this era, ballet was forming its aesthetic identity. In the early 1800s, the Paris Operá Ballet sought to create pink tights, because bare legs were too risqué for Parisians to view.[6] The concept of *ballet pink* complimented the all-white company's skin tone. Additionally, in the 1800s was the *ballet blanc*, a phrase used to describe the traditional white, soft, bell-shaped tutus that reach the calf or ankle. These tutus were designed by Eugène Lami for Italian dancer Marie Taglioni in the ballets *La Sylphide* and *Giselle* among others to support the ethereal nature of her roles. Ballet blanc was originally created to embody ethereal dance roles, but like the ballet pink, it would eventually be used as the underpinnings of racial exclusivity in the field.

In Russia, *Orientalism* and racialized ideologies were prominent in choreographies such as *The Nutcracker*. This ballet was adopted from Prussian Ernst Theodor Hoffman's book, *The Nutcracker and the Mouse King* (1816). Years later in December of 1892, composer Pyotr Ilyich Tchaikovsky collaborated with choreographers Marcus Petipa and then Lev Ivanov to create *The Nutcracker* ballet which premiered in St. Petersburg, Russia, at the Mariinsky Theatre.[7] Today, *The Nutcracker* is performed in thousands of theaters around the globe at Christmas time and has become a major holiday tradition. *The Nutcracker* holds gendered and racialized roles while inappropriately displaying "traditional" cultural customs – caricatures of Black, Latinx, and Asian communities as seen in its Arabian, Coffee, and Chinese variations. *The Nutcracker* is only one example of racialized ideologies and practices within Russian ballet.

In the 1890s, impresario Serge Diaghilev began curating visual art exhibits and performances. In 1909, Diaghilev formed the Ballets Russes. He worked with composer Igor Stravinsky, and did not follow the style of ballet blanc; instead, they engaged with the image of the "harem dancer" by creating exoticized ballets such as *Schéhérazade* (1909), *Les*

*Orientales* (1910), *The Firebird* (1910), and *Petrushka* (1911).[8] These ballets captured how Europeans imagined Eastern cultures to be. Their images seldom coincided with reality, rather they encapsulated Orientalist aesthetics and racialized stereotypes in order to feed European audiences' demand for exotic images of faraway lands.[9] The critic Valerian Svetlov (1860–1935) wrote ecstatically: "the first season of the Diaghilev Ballet must be commemorated in letters of gold in the annals of Russian Ballet. To say it was successful is to say nothing. It was a revelation, a major event in the artistic life of Paris."[10] Diaghilev and his team drew upon racialized stereotypes that satisfied Parisian audiences' ideologies and assumptions of an exotic fantasy Orient. Particularly in Ballets Russes' *Schéhérazade*, in the violent, sexualized, and interracial depictions of the ballet were contingent on their exotic location of Persia and made this ballet a success.[11] Choreographer Michel Fokine addresses the Orientalism within *Schéhérazade*:

> After the composition of this ballet, I undertook the study of authentic Oriental dances. But nothing would have induced me to stage my ballet in the authentic Oriental style, for such an undertaking would have required a genuine Oriental orchestra. The symphonic music of Rimsky-Korsakov would be completely unsuited. The Orient, based on authentic Arabic, Persian, and Hindu movements, was still the Orient of the imagination. Dancers with bare feet, performing mostly with their arms and torsos, constituted a concept far removed from the Oriental ballet of the time.[12]

These racialized assumptions appeased the Parisian audience and created a new desire and genre for oriental style repertoires that Ballets Russes understood and continued to produce.

Diaghilev worked with composers Maurice Ravel and Claude Debussy and fashion designers Coco Chanel and Léon Baskt. He also brought painters to design vivid theatrical backdrops and sets including Pablo Picasso and Henri Matisse. Diaghilev employed Russian ballerina Anna

Pavlova, young choreographers George Balanchine and Mikhail Fokine and the luminary male dancer and choreographer of the time Vaslav Nijinky.[13] Diaghilev's death would signify the end of the Ballets Russes, but it would maintain its legacy as the leading company of ballet modernity.[14]

## THE "CLASSICAL BLACK" ERA

As ballet in the 20th century progressed, ballet dancing in Broadway shows was often eclipsed by tap dancing and ballroom dance. In the early 1900s, Mikhail Mordkin, a Russian dancer, partnered with Anna Pavlova and the Ballets Russes to perform at the Metropolitan Opera House.[15] This would give America its first glimpse of ballet as an artform. However, Black dancers were excluded from many dance studios and ballet spaces, because of Black Codes and racial exclusionary laws such as the Jim Crow Laws. This resulted in Black people creating their own spaces to introduce Black children to ballet. In 1929, Essie Marie Dorsey founded the first dance studio in Philadelphia to offer ballet classes for Black children. Dorsey also offered tap, ballroom, and acrobatics, allowing Black children formal dance training in a variety of styles. Essie Marie Dorsey and Thomas Cannon, a principal dancer of Littlefield Ballet Company, both taught at the school which was sponsored by W.E.B. Du Bois's symposium "The Negro in Art."[16] Du Bois believed that the emerging proliferation of art throughout the 1920s gave rise to a new spirit within the Black community and ignited this *renaissance* by creating a generation of Black artistic creatives which was a part of the "New Negro" movement, known today as the **Harlem Renaissance**.[17]

## DANCING THROUGH BALLET HISTORY TO TODAY

After World War I and the Russian Revolution, many Russian dancers and choreographers immigrated to the United States; George Balanchine being one of them.

Despite the fact that the *Classical Black* era had begun to take place in the early 1900s, predominantly white choreographers such as George Balanchine and British born Antony Tudor were coined as the pioneers of American ballet.[18] In 1934, Balanchine came to the United States and met Lincoln Kirstein – a novelist, poet, critic, and philanthropist.[19] Together they founded American Ballet, which is now called the School of American Ballet (SAB).

Also, during this time, American Ballet Theatre (ABT) was founded in 1939, by Lucia Chase, Richard Pleasant, and Oliver Smith in New York City. They had their inaugural season in 1940 and included the works of 11 choreographers including Mikhail Fokine and Antony Tudor and American dancer and choreographer Agnes de Mille.[20] De Mille choreographed their world premiere entitled Black Ritual (Obeah). This ballet was performed by 16 Black women, none of whom were named in the program.[21] Not acknowledging the names of these dancers punctuated the racialized exclusion within ballet and minimized the contributions of Black dancers. In a review by *New York Amsterdam News*, Dan Burley, the pianist and music critic, who was a Black man, noted, "It was the first time in the history of the ballet in New York that Negroes have been included in the theatre's repertory."[22] This isolated ballet was only performed three times. After this season, Agnes de Mille featured a few Black dancers, when working for American Ballet Theatre onward, without hiring them to be a part of the company; dancers included Carmen de Lavallade and Judith Jamison who both performed in de Mille's production of "The Four Mary's" and danced for Alvin Ailey American Dance Theater.[23]

In 1955, Arthur Mitchell, a dark-skinned Black man from Harlem, who danced with confidence and an unmatched physical artistry, was invited by both Lincoln Kirstein and George Balanchine to join New York City Ballet. He was the first Black dancer at the company, and within a year he was promoted to principal. In 1957, Mitchell debuted his principal role in Balanchine's premiere of *Agon*. Mitchell was paired with white ballerina Diana Adams to perform this intertwining *pas de deux*. Their duet created a tense stir with the audience because, up until this point, Black male dancers were not allowed to be in close contact with white women on stage.[24] This was just two years after 14-year-old Emmitt Till was lynched in Mississippi after being accused of offending a white woman in a grocery story.[25] Separation laws were still very much intact and Balanchine's casting choice challenged racial segregation. Arthur Mitchell experienced a lot of racism while at the company in which many parents did not want Arthur Mitchell (a Black man) partnering their daughters. An audience member even yelled "Oh, my God! They have a nigger in the company!" during his debut performance, and television stations refused to show Mitchell partnering Diana Adams in *Agon*, but that did not stop Arthur Mitchell as he continued dancing with the company.[26]

Also, during the 1950s, two Black women by the names of Janet Collins and Raven Wilkinson broke barriers for Black women in ballet. Both Janet Collins and Raven Wilkinson endured various forms of racism and discrimination. Janet Collins was the first Black artist, of any discipline, to perform at the Metropolitan Opera House. She was also the first prima ballerina to be contracted for the Metropolitan Opera Ballet. Collins was vocal about the discrimination and racism that took place within ballet. She shared in her biography that when she auditioned for the Ballets Russes de Monte-Carlo she was told that that she had to perform with make-up to make her skin lighter and she refused.[27] Artistic director Zachary Solov invited Collins to dance with the Metropolitan Opera Ballet in which she became the first Black ballerina. She performed with the Metropolitan Opera Ballet through 1954 until she left for a successful solo career in which she toured the United States and Canada.[28]

Raven Wilkinson became the first Black dancer to be part of a major ballet company that stands alone, as a company, and not as an extension of an opera house – The Ballets Russes de Monte-Carlo. Contrasting Collins, Wilkinson accepted the invite with The Ballets Russes and often lightened her skin with make-up for performances. However, she refused to hide her identity if asked directly, despite other non-Black dancers advising Wilkinson to say she was Spanish given her fair complexion.[29] Wilkinson toured through Europe and the United States with the company. When she reached the United States, she encountered extreme racism. In Montgomery, Alabama, while at her hotel, Wilkinson encountered a Ku Klux Klan convention in the same hotel. She and the Artistic Director felt that it would not be safe for her to perform that evening. Following this incident, Wilkinson returned home to New York City and took a hiatus from dancing. It wasn't until 1973 that she joined the Dutch National Ballet and continued a successful career until her semi-retirement in 1985.[30]

In the 1960s, Arthur Mitchell transitioned out of New York City Ballet, and began to guest perform for other companies internationally. In 1968 Mitchell was en route to the airport to go to Brazil where he had been invited to form a new dance company when he received the devastating news that Dr. Martin Luther King Jr. had been assassinated. Mitchell understood that dance could be a strong social justice force, so he decided to stay in America and create a space for Black people to practice ballet in New York City. With Karel Shook, the former ballet master of the Dutch National Ballet, he founded the Dance Theatre of Harlem in 1969. In the basement of a church in Harlem, New York, Dance Theatre of Harlem (DTH) became a safe space for Black dancers and dancers of color thus creating much needed cultural inclusion within ballet. Mitchell took experienced dancers and dancers with little to no training and built a company that exhibited Black dancers doing ballet. Mitchell utilized his experience with New York City Ballet and transcended it through Dance Theatre of Harlem with performances such as *Agon* in which starred Lydia Abarca and Mel Tomlinson. Mitchell invited Lydia Abarca – a girl from Harlem who just enjoyed dancing but had very limited training and interest in ballet, to become a founding member for DTH. She accepted and became his muse. She was not only the first principal dancer at DTH but the first Black woman to be a principal dancer in a major company in the United States. She was photographed by Lord Snowdon – a

British photographer and filmmaker who married Princess Margaret, the sister of Queen Elizabeth. Lord Snowdon followed Abarca through 152nd street in Harlem, New York, as she walked to ballet. He then took photographs at DTH with the company and through his photography he captured Dance Theatre of Harlem and the essence of Black ballet dancers. As time continued, DTH "became the first African American classical-ballet company to achieve international acclaim as a neoclassical ballet company."[31] The company toured South Africa after apartheid and the Soviet Union.[32]

DTH reconsidered classical ballets by giving them a uniquely African American perspective. This made their repertoire more relatable to their intended audience – Black people who lived within the community of Harlem. In 1984, Frederic Franklin – an American ballet dancer and director, restaged the original *Giselle* and created *Creole Giselle* for the DTH. It starred Virginia Johnson as Giselle Lanaux – a young woman from Louisiana in the 1940s and, as one critic stated, the performance was "critically acclaimed in both London and New York for its transfer of ballet into the Creole ambiance of 19th-century Louisiana."[33] *Creole Giselle* reclaimed a classical ballet that had historically been an exclusive ballet blanc production. He even changed the costumes and created a silk shift that was used by the entire corps de ballet and principal female dancers opposed to the traditional Romantic tutu. DTH continued to challenge the concept of ballet blanc as well as the idea of solely wearing ballet pink. In the early 1970s, one of Mitchell's founding members, Llanchie Stevenson, now known as Aminah L. Ahmad became the influence behind Mitchell's adoption of flesh-tone tights and shoes which he debuted in the 1970s. Prior to DTH, Stevenson danced with Radio City Music Hall as the first Black member of the corps de ballet. She then received a scholarship to study with the School of American Ballet for two years. After two years, Stevenson noticed that her peers were being offered contracts and when she inquired about her standing with the company, Diana Adams, the Dean of the School of American Ballet, told Stevenson that Balanchine was not ready to "break the corps color line" by having a Black woman in the corps de ballet, even though he had Arthur Mitchell, a Black male dancer in the company already. The intersectionality of race and gender play a role in the experiences of Black women in classical ballet.

After Stevenson left SAB, she then went to the National Ballet of Washington. After dancing for a few years with National Ballet of Washington as a corps de ballet member, Mitchell asked Stevenson to become a member of his company DTH. She accepted and joined as a founding member of DTH. During DTH's European tour, Stevenson started wearing flesh-tone tights over her pink tights because she states, "I noticed that my arms were a different color than my legs, I thought that I looked disjointed." Once wearing flesh-tone tights, Stevenson realized that flesh-tone also made her look slimmer. After wearing her flesh-tone tights for a little while, Arthur Mitchell noticed and liked the idea and so he then decided to have everyone within the company wear flesh-tone tights. Throughout Stevenson's time touring and performing with DTH, she noticed that she was not being cast in the roles she wanted, despite being a principal dancer for the company, and she felt that her lack of roles was due to her weight. She began reading a book titled, *How to Eat to Live* by Elijah Muhammad to help her lose weight. Through the inspiration of this book, she became interested in the Islamic faith and after reading about Allah in Muhammad's book she started attending meetings for the Nation of Islam. Shortly afterwards, she retired from DTH and converted to Islam which is why she changed her name to Aminah Ahmad. Throughout Stevenson's career, she became the catalyst behind flesh-toned tights for Black ballerinas. During this time, flesh-toned tights and pointe shoes became an act of emancipation over the racial exclusion that the ballet blanc and ballet pink standards had upheld for over 100 years. They also demonstrated that these changes for inclusivity can be made without changing the art of ballet.[34]

This racialized declaration for flesh-toned tights transcended through the 1980s and 1990s when Lauren Anderson – the first Black principal dancer at Houston Ballet made it a point to wear tights and pointe shoes that complimented her darker skin. Growing up in Houston, Texas, Anderson was inspired by Dance Theatre of Harlem and loved seeing them perform. She states,

> when I turned about 9, I saw my first Black ballerina. My mom took me to see Dance Theatre of Harlem here at Jones Hall in Houston, Texas and I couldn't believe it. I was like 'Oh my gosh!' They were doing a Balanchine piece and there was one Black ballerina and then another one ran across and then another one ran across and then I turned to my mom and said there's a whole stage of Black ballet dancers.... Then, every time Dance Theatre of Harlem came, we would go see them.

The influence, and representation of DTH transcended through her and artistic director Ben Stevenson (not related to Llanchie Stevenson) played a role regarding Anderson's advocacy for wearing flesh-tone tights.[35]

This influence and advocacy also transcended through Precious Adams, an African American dancer who currently dances for English National Ballet. In 2018, Adams made a statement that she would no longer perform on stage wearing pink tights and would wear brown tights that complimented her skin tone. She states,

> It changes the aesthetic – you want there to be a continuation between your upper and lower body and there's a big disconnect if I put pink tights on.... I want to look my best on stage. I think it [pink tights] ruins the line of my body.

Adams also shared that in 2011, she studied at the Bolshoi Ballet Academy in Moscow and was the first Black woman to graduate from Bolshoi. During her time at the Bolshoi Ballet Academy, she faced racial discrimination which led her to be left out of performances, prevented from auditions and was even told to "try and rub the Black off." She left Bolshoi Ballet Academy in 2014 and was a two-time Prix de Lausanne winner in Switzerland before joining the English National Ballet where she danced along with Black male dancer Brooklyn Mack who was a guest artist at the time.

The declaration for flesh-toned tights captures a shift in the ballet aesthetic identity in which the aesthetic attire does not completely change but just becomes more racially inclusive to reflect the array of skin tones that are included in ballet.

Also, from the early 2000s onward, the conversations around race and ballet began to shift and were different from the trend and conversation of Orientalism that took place in the early 1800s regarding the repertoires being created. Misty Copeland began using her platform, as a ballet dancer, to discuss race and racism against actual dancers within ballet. In 2012, Copeland began surfacing major headlines when she starred as a soloist, in ABT's premiere of the *Firebird* (2012). She shares with *USA Today*,

> My first performance of *Firebird* in New York City was a really, really special night and a very important season for me. I was still a soloist (when I was given) that role at American Ballet Theatre, and the audience was full of brown people for the first time ever. I could open people's eyes and minds to what was possible in terms of diversifying –not just the dancers on stage, but the people in the audience.[36]

Copeland became a soloist in 2007 and a member of the corps de ballet since 2001. Throughout her career she became vocal about race and racism within ballet and her background as not the "conventional" ballerina given her upbringing and starting ballet at the age of 13 years old. In 2015, during ABT's 75th anniversary, Copeland was promoted to principal dancer making her the first Black woman to be a principal dancer at ABT. She became a widely known activist bringing the conversation of race and ballet to the mainstream public eye and being very vocal about the ballet industry being more inclusive.

## CONCLUSION

The fight and advocacy for racial justice in ballet continues. There are systemic changes that must occur. As Gia Koulas asked in her article "Where are All the Black Swans?" there is still a need for more Black occupancy amongst dancers as well as higher administrative positions. In 2020 alone, Black male dancers Calvin Royal III and Gabe Shayer have been promoted to principal and soloist within American Ballet Theatre. Former New York City Ballet dancer Aesha Ash became the first Black woman permanent faculty member at School of American Ballet and former New York City Ballet member Andrea Long-Naidu became a faculty member for Boston Ballet. As we move forward, we are seeing how this conversation of racial justice is creating opportunities for more inclusion without changing the technique that has been codified hundreds of years before.

As I continue my journey of filling the gaps of where all of the Black dancers reside within the canon of dance history, I am constantly learning and expanding this history as ballet continues to become more inclusive. In the future, I hope this chapter can be expanded to share more stories and historical moments that will inspire young dancers who may have felt, or who currently feel, excluded from ballet; and I hope they are now able to not just dream of a mysterious Black ballerina (as I did) but can actually see an array of Black ballet dancers and feel inspired and accepted into this ballet world.

## FURTHER READING

### Films:

*Black Ballerina Documentary* https://blackballerinadocumentary.org
*Black Ballerina* shares stories of Black women of several generations who became ballerinas. They share their racialized experiences and how they continue to challenge the racial stereotypes used to exclude Black women from ballet.
*A Ballerina's Tale Documentary*
*A Ballerina's Tale* provides a behind-the-scenes of Misty Copeland and the triumphs and struggles that she and dancers before her experience as Black women in ballet.

## Books:

Au, Susan. "Ballet and Modern Dance." *ASSESSMENT* 1, no. 2 (1974): 3. *Ballet and Modern Dance* provides a historical guide to ballet and modern dance from Medici to Manhattan, New York. Au provides a foundation in which she highlights significant historical moments and people throughout the dance world.

Gaiser, Carrie. "Caught Dancing: Hybridity, Stability, and Subversion in Dance Theatre of Harlem's Creole 'Giselle'." *Theatre Journal* (2006): 269–289. "Caught Dancing: Hybridity, Stability, and Subversion in Dance Theatre of Harlem's Creole 'Giselle'" examines Dance Theatre of Harlem's production of *Creole Giselle* and elaborates on the conjunction of Black dancing bodies and European classical ballet style techniques. This article provides additional information on racial and cultural negotiations within ballet.

Gottschild, Brenda. *The black dancing body: A geography from coon to cool.* Springer, 2016.
*The black dancing body* provides a chronological map of Black bodies throughout a variety of different dance genres. Gottschild addresses the influence and importance of Black bodies throughout dance history which has historically been omitted from many dance history literatures.

Lewin, Yaël Tamar, and Janet Collins. *Night's dancer: the life of Janet Collins.* Wesleyan University Press, 2011. *Night's dancer: the life of Janet Collins* is a biography about Janet Collins and how she broke barriers as the first Black woman to be a prima ballerina. This book provides an in-depth insight into the racialized experience of Janet Collins in ballet.

# TIMELINE

Late 1300s–1400s – Ballet is created in Italy.

1533 – Catherine de Medici moves to France, bringing *ballet de cour* or ballet of the court.

1661 – Louis XIV forms the Académie Royale de Danse, the first state funded school for ballet.

1689 – Ballet reaches Moscow.

1776 – The Bolshoi Ballet is founded.

Early 1800s – Romantic era of ballet begins, with notable performances such as *Giselle*.

1909 – Serge Diaghilev forms the Ballets Russes.

1934 – George Balanchine and Lincoln Kirstein founded American Ballet, now called the School of American Ballet (SAB).

1939 – American Ballet Theatre (ABT) is founded by Lucia Chase, Richard Pleasant, and Oliver Smith in New York City.

1955 – Arthur Mitchell joins New York City Ballet.

1969 – Arthur Mitchell and Karel Shook founded the Dance Theatre of Harlem.

Early 1970s – Dance Theatre of Harlem starts wearing flesh-tone tights.

1975 – Lydia Abarca became the first Black ballerina to appear on the cover of *Dance Magazine*.

1982 – Debra Austin became the first Black principal dancer promoted at Pennsylvania Ballet.

1990 – Lauren Anderson became the first Black principal dancer at Houston Ballet and continued the racialized declaration of wearing flesh-tone tights.

2015 – Misty Copeland becomes the first Black principal dancer at ABT on their 75th Anniversary.

# REFERENCES

Allen, Zita. "Arthur Mitchell: The Man and His Legacy," 2018. http://amsterdamnews.com/news/2018/sep/27/arthur-mitchell-man-and-his-legacy/.

Anderson, Jack. "Sallie Wilson, Keeper Of the Tudor Flame." *The New York Times*. 1992. www.nytimes.com/1992/05/24/arts/dance-sallie-wilson-keeper-of-the-tudor-flame.html.

"Arthur Mitchell, a Dancer Who Broke Down Barriers, Brings Archive to Columbia." *Columbia Magazine*, 2015. https://magazine.columbia.edu/article/arthur-mitchell-dancer-who-broke-down-barriers-brings-archive-columbia.

DaCosta Johnson, Djassi. "Dance Theatre of Harlem." *Kinfolk*, Volume 23. 2017. www.kinfolk.com/dance-theatre-of-harlem/.

Fokine, Michel. *Fokine, Memoirs of a Ballet Master*. London: Costable, 1961.

Fuhrer, Margaret. "Raven Wilkinson's Extraordinary Life: An Exclusive Interview." *Pointe*. 2014. www.pointemagazine.com/raven-wilkinson-interview-2412812564.html.

Gaiser, Carrie. "Caught Dancing: Hybridity, Stability, and Subversion in Dance Theatre of Harlem's Creole 'Giselle'." *Theatre Journal.* 2006: 269–289.

Genné, Beth. "Glorifying the American Woman: Josephine Baker and George Balanchine." *Discourses in Dance* 3, no. 1. 2005: 31–57.

Gottschild, Brenda Dixon. "But Black is Beautiful! 1950s–1980s." In *Joan Myers Brown & the Audacious Hope of the Black Ballerina*, pp. 91–134. Palgrave Macmillan, New York, 2012.

Grigoriev, S.L. *The Diaghilev Ballet, 1909–1929.* NY: Constable, 1953.

Homans, Jennifer. *Apollo's Angels: A History of Ballet.* New York: Random House, 2010.

Howard, Theresa Ruth. "Is Classical Ballet Ready to Embrace Flesh-Tone Tights?" *Dance Magazine.* 2018. www.dancemagazine.com/ballet-flesh-tone-tights-2612825762.html.

Jackson, La'Toya Princess. 2019. *Black Swans Shattering the Glass Ceiling: A Historical Perspective the Evolution of Historically Black Ballet Companies—From Katherine Dunham to Arthur Mitchell.* Diss.

Keely, Dominic. "A History of Ballet in Russia," 2017. www.scenic.co.uk/news/a-history-of-ballet-in-russia.

Keller, Bill. 1992. "Harlem Dance Theater Testing South Africa." *The New York Times*, September 21. Accessed on August 8, 2018. www.nytimes.com/1992/09/21/arts/harlem-dance-theater-testing-south-africa.html.

Lansky, Chava Pearl. "Remembering Raven Wilkinson, Trailblazing Ballerina." *Pointe Magazine.* 2018. www.pointemagazine.com/remembering-raven-wilkinson-trailblazing-black-ballerina-2623864149.html.

Lewin, Yaël Tamar, and Janet Collins. *Night's dancer: the life of Janet Collins.* Wesleyan University Press, 2011.

Lifar, Serge. *Serge Diaghilev.* Read Books Ltd, 2011.

Lozynsky, Artem. "AND THE BALLETS RUSSES." *Situations*1. 2007.

Maher, Erin K. "Ballet, Race, and Agnes de Mille's Black Ritual." *The Musical Quarterly* 97, no. 3. 2014: 390–428.

Needham, Maureen. "Louis xiv and the Académie Royale de Danse, 1661—A commentary and translation." *Dance Chronicle* 20, no. 2. 1997: 173–190.

Norman, Larry. The theatrical Baroque: European Plays, Painting and Poetry. The University of Chicago Library. 2001.

Paydar, Nikoo. "Exploiting Russian and Oriental Stereotypes: The Ballets Russes Schéhérazade in Paris, 1910." *Artl@s Bulletin* 2, no. 1 2013: 4.

Robinson, Sekani L. "Black Swans: Black Female Ballet Dancers and the Management of Emotional and Aesthetic Labor." PhD diss., UC Santa Barbara, 2018.

Scholl, Tim. *From Petipa to Balanchine: Classical Revival and the Modernisation of Ballet.* Routledge, 2003.

Scott Michael. "The Harlem Renaissance: Black Cultural Innovation Unleashed." Libertarianism.org. 2020. www.libertarianism.org/ articles/harlem-renaissance-black-cultural-innovation-unleashed.

Stevenson, Llanchie. MOBBallet.org. (2021, January 2). https:// mobballet.org/index.php/2017/12/27/llanchie-stevenson/.

Taylor, Burton. "How the Creole 'Giselle' Took Form." 1984. www.nytimes.com/1984/10/14/arts/how-the-creole-giselle-took-form.html.

Thurber, Jon. "Janet Collins, 86; Broke Ballet Color Line." Los Angeles Times. June 2, 2003. www.latimes.com/archives/ la-xpm-2003-jun-02-me-collins2-story.html.

Wiley, Roland John. 1985. *Tchaikovsky's ballets: Swan Lake, Sleeping Beauty, Nutcracker.* Oxford: Clarendon Press.

# NOTES

1 Maureen Needham, "Louis XIV and the Académie Royale de Danse, 1661—A commentary and translation," *Dance Chronicle* 20, no. 2. 1997: 173–190; There were three different academics that were a part of the academy and Pierre Beauchamps was the one who invented the system that Raoul Auger Reuillet used, and more than 325 dances and repertoires have been notated within this system which is how we have classic repertoires documented today. Also, Beauchamps is credited for codifying the basic five positions that are still used today all of which are sequential teaching methods (Needham, 1997, 175).

2 Needham, 1997, 176; The thirteen experts were rewarded as members of the royal household and exempted from certain taxes and the ballet masters were receiving a generous number of profits for their lessons as well. Needham, 1997, 174, 176.

3 Needham, 1997, 174, 176.

4 Needham, 1997, 174, 176.

5 Artem Lozynsky, "AND THE BALLETS RUSSES," *Situations* 1, 2007.

6 Pointe shoes were created in the 1820s and while the very first pointe shoes were white, they quickly became pink to "match" the tights to create longer lines with the dancer's body.

7 Roland John Wiley, *Tchaikovsky's ballets: Swan Lake, Sleeping Beauty, Nutcracker* (Oxford: Clarendon Press, 1985).

8   Lozynsky, "AND THE BALLETS RUSSES," 2007.

9   The romantic ballerina symbolizing the "soul" of the West rose on her toes, as the "harem dancer" representing the "body" of the East sank to the floor.

10  S.L. Grigoriev, *The Diaghilev Ballet, 1909–1929* (NY: Constable, 1953), 25–26.

11  Nikoo Paydar, "Exploiting Russian and Oriental Stereotypes: The Ballets Russes Schéhérazade in Paris, 1910," *Artl@s Bulletin* 2, no. 1. 2013: 4.

12  Michel Fokine, *Fokine, Memoirs of a Ballet Master* (London: Costable, 1961).

13  Serge Lifar, *Serge Diaghilev* (Read Books Ltd, 2011).

14  Tim Scholl, *From Petipa to Balanchine: Classical Revival and the Modernisation of Ballet.* (Routledge, 2003).

15  Anna Pavlova danced with the Ballets Russes briefly. She went with Diaghilev to Paris where he signed her for his first Paris performance in 1909. In 1910, she formed her own company with eight Russian dancers and then in 1913, she toured America and other countries for the next 15 years (www.russianballethistory.com/annapavlovathelegend.htm);   Jennifer Homans, *Apollo's Angels: A History of Ballet* (New York: Random House, 2010), 450.

16  Brenda Dixon Gottschild, "But Black is Beautiful! 1950s–1980s," In *Joan Myers Brown & the Audacious Hope of the Black Ballerina*, ed. Palgrave Macmillan (New York, 2012), 91–134.

17  Michael Scott, "The Harlem Renaissance: Black Cultural Innovation Unleashed," Libertarianism.org, 2020. www.libertarianism.org/articles/harlem-renaissance-black-cultural-innovation-unleashed; Harlem Renaissance which was a time of revival for intellectual and cultural Black music, art, fashion, dance, theater, literature, and politics. It was centered in Harlem, New York and was the time of Langston Hughes, Zora Neale Hurston, Alain Locke, and many other Black creatives (Scott, 2020).

18  La'Toya Princess Jackson, 2019, *Black Swans Shattering the Glass Ceiling: A Historical Perspective the Evolution of Historically Black Ballet Companies—From Katherine Dunham to Arthur Mitchell.* Diss.

19  Given Lincoln Kirstein's social justice work, he envisioned desegregating ballet as well as moving away from its elitist ideals. The idea was to "take four white girls and four white boys [four Black girls and four Black boys] – about sixteen years old and eight of the same, [Black]" to create a number titled *Two Faced Woman* which would be a fusion of Black and white dancers, however this vision was not fulfilled.

20  Jack Anderson, "Sallie Wilson, Keeper Of the Tudor Flame." *The New York Times.* 1992. www.nytimes.com/1992/05/24/arts/dance-sallie-wilson-keeper-of-the-tudor-flame.html; British Antony Tudor was similar to Balanchine in which they

both extended range and variety within their vision of ballet, which made them influential to American Ballet and American Ballet style. Tudor was inspired to dance after watching Pavlova and the Diaghilev Ballet and while Balanchine placed emphasis on the extroversion of his dancers, Tudor focused on the direct expression of personal feelings (Anderson, 1992).

21 Their names being Carole Ash, Maudelle Bass, Valerie Black, Clementina Collingwood, Muriel Cook, Mable Hart, Edith Hurd, Anne Jones, Lawuane Kennard, Evelyn Pilcher, Edith Ross, Elizabeth Thompson, Dorothy Williams, Lavinia Williams, and Bernice Willis.

22 Erin K. Maher, "Ballet, Race, and Agnes de Mille's Black Ritual," *The Musical Quarterly* 97, no. 3. 2014: 390.

23 Sekani L. Robinson, "Black Swans: Black Female Ballet Dancers and the Management of Emotional and Aesthetic Labor," PhD diss., UC Santa Barbara, 2018.

24 Beth Genné, "Glorifying the American Woman: Josephine Baker and George Balanchine," *Discourses in Dance* 3, no. 1. 2005: 31–57.

25 In 1955, Emmitt Till was accused of offending a white woman – Carolyn Bryant – in her family's grocery store in which case he was lynched and later Bryant confessed that she fabricated the testimony.

26 Zita Allen, "Arthur Mitchell: The Man and His Legacy," 2018, http://amsterdamnews.com/news/2018/sep/27/arthur-mitchell-man-and-his-legacy/.

27 Yaël Tamar Lewin and Janet Collins, *Night's dancer: the life of Janet Collins* (Wesleyan University Press, 2011).

28 Jon Thurber, "Janet Collins, 86; Broke Ballet Color Line," *Los Angeles Times* June 2, 2003. www.latimes.com/archives/la-xpm-2003-jun-02-me-collins2-story.html.

29 Chava Pearl Lansky, "Remembering Raven Wilkinson, Trailblazing Ballerina," *Pointe Magazine*, 2018, www.pointemagazine.com/remembering-raven-wilkinson-trailblazing-black-ballerina-2623864149.html.

30 Margaret Fuhrer, "Raven Wilkinson's Extraordinary Life: An Exclusive Interview," *Pointe*, 2014, www.pointemagazine.com/raven-wilkinson-interview-2412812564.html.

31 Columbia Magazine, "Arthur Mitchell, a Dancer Who Broke Down Barriers, Brings Archive to Columbia," 2015, https://magazine.columbia.edu/article/arthur-mitchell-dancer-who-broke-down-barriers-brings-archive-columbia.

32 Bill Keller, "Harlem Dance Theater Testing South Africa," *The New York Times*, September 21, 1992, Accessed on August 8, 2018, www.nytimes.com/1992/09/21/arts/harlem-dance-theater-testing-south-africa.html.

33 Carrie Gaiser, "Caught Dancing: Hybridity, Stability, and Subversion in Dance Theatre of Harlem's Creole 'Giselle'," *Theatre Journal*, 2006: 269–289; Burton Taylor,

"How the Creole 'Giselle' Took Form," 1984, www.nytimes.com/1984/10/14/arts/how-the-creole-giselle-took-form.html.

34 *Llanchie Stevenson*, MOBBallet.org, (2021, January 2), https://mobballet.org/index.php/2017/12/27/llanchie-stevenson/.

35 Ben Stevenson noticed that Anderson's legs appeared grey under the lights in pink tights and so they decided to test a few shades of brown tights but were not having any success and so Stevenson said, "Call Dance Theatre of Harlem and find out what they use" and from there, there was no going back to pink tights for Anderson.

36 S. Hutcheson, *How I became a ballerina: Misty Copeland, USA Today*, www.usatoday.com/story/money/careers/2020/03/31/how-misty-copeland-became-principal-dancer-american-ballet-theatre/2929620001/.

CHAPTER 5

# Modern and Postmodern Dance
## War and Choreography in the 20th and 21st Centuries

*Kate Mattingly*

Have you ever looked at an image and seen it switch or become something else? One of the most famous examples of this kind of ambiguous figure is "Rubin's Vase," which shows an outline of a symmetrical vase or two human profiles facing each other, depending on how you see the background and the object [see Figure 5.1]. This image is named for Edgar John Rubin, a Danish psychologist and phenomenologist, who developed this concept in 1915; in Rubin's words,

> When two fields have a common border, and one is seen as figure and the other as ground, the immediate perceptual experience is characterized by a shaping effect which emerges from the common border of the fields and which operates only on one field or operates more strongly on one than on the other.[1]

In other words, when we, as viewers, flip or shift what we consider ground or background with what we consider figure or object, we can interpret images and borders in different ways.

What do ambiguous figures have to do with dance history? When we examine the background or conditions that nurtured artists during the 20th century, we notice important relationships between global conflicts and genres of dance. By considering the impact of wars and uprisings on how values and identities are formed, we see how and why certain art-

DOI: 10.4324/9781003185918-5

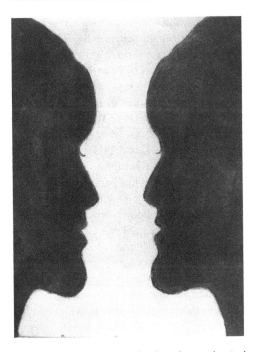

**Figure 5.1:** Image drawn for this chapter by Catherine Long

ists became the canonical choreographers of dance history. This attention to background and figure, or conditions and choreographers, is not often found in the writing of history, which has tended to make a priority of bracketing certain choreographers and performances, and focusing on aesthetic characteristics, personal biographies, and creative processes. By widening our lens on the environments that surround dancers, and how their work is filtered through the writing of critics and historians, we can trace the contours of their artistic projects as figures against the background of global conflict.

This chapter focuses on three performances created in the 20th and 21st centuries to show how artists respond to global conflicts, uphold nationalistic ideals, and challenge hegemonic identities. I am using the word nationalistic to encompass two approaches: first, choreography that reflects a particular image of a country, its peoples' hopes, interests, and longings, and second, the values of a nation that can be ascertained from the ways certain genres and performances are leveraged on behalf of a nation.[2] The performance *Appalachian Spring* (1944), created by Martha Graham with music by Aaron Copland and set design by Isamu Noguchi, is analyzed as exemplifying "modern dance." It was first performed at the Library of Congress in Washington D.C., across the street from the U.S. Capitol. Merce Cunningham's *RainForest* (1968) with music by David Tudor, set design by Andy Warhol, and costumes by Jasper Johns, is analyzed as a "postmodern" performance. It was first performed at Buffalo State College, offering us a view of how higher education, historically and currently, promotes certain dance genres and choreographic approaches. *Memoirs of Active Service* (2006), choreographed by Maaka Pepene for Atamira Dance Company, is described as a contemporary performance that reconfigures definitions of nationalism by emphasizing interdependence and connection. A recent interview conducted with Jack Gray, Atamira's current director, provides insights into relationships among dancers, identities, and histories.

Rather than impose a linear chronology on dance history, I selected these three moments to show how artists respond to cultural priorities at distinct historical moments. These three performances offer a way to take a temperature and note continuities and discontinuities across geographies and eras. While I associate these individual performances with the categories "modern," "postmodern," and "contemporary" dance, I am aware that any label – including "modern," "postmodern," "contemporary" – is fraught because it imposes a sense of coherence or unity on artistic practices that can differ immensely. It is also important to keep in mind the networks of support that undergird any artist's endeavors, and these include funders, critics, patrons, and collaborators. For instance, in my analysis of Graham's work, I include her association with critic John Martin, his defining of modern dance, and Graham's own writing about dance as an American art in the years between World Wars I and II. An ambiguous figure is a resonant image for this analysis because it is often depicted in black-and-white and, similarly, dance history in the United States is often presented as a segregated narrative that separates white dance forms and their codified techniques from Black artistry and innovation. Often the knowledge systems and art forms of Indigenous and Asian cultures are left out of these histories.[3] This chapter addresses and challenges these gaps by calling attention to the pernicious impacts of settler colonialism and racism in histories of nations as well as dance.

Ultimately, I ask you, as a reader, how do today's global conflicts and crises influence your engagement with dance as an art form? More specifically, how do these global events influence the perspectives and value systems you bring to engaging with artists? Do you perceive their performances as being in dialog with – or a response to – current events? A brilliant choreographer, Bill T. Jones, once said that all performances are political, even the ones the artists themselves think of as apolitical. In his own words, Jones said,

> I think it's impossible to perform any ritualized activity in a public sphere that is politically neutral.... Merce [Cunningham] claims that it's politically neutral. It's not. Trisha [Brown] who is a teacher to me, who I love, thinks it's politically neutral. It's not.[4]

While the three examples I have chosen slant this analysis towards events happening in the United States and Aotearoa,[5] also known as New Zealand, my argument can be applied to other regions and countries: how do historical and current choreographers reflect the ethos of an era? Do you find their performances to be in dialog with dominant or marginalized identities, ideas, or cultures? What is foregrounded in their work, or made the figure, and what happens when we bring the background into focus, noticing its conditions and contours? We can apply this method to any performance, and to any analysis of the ways eras become historicized, starting with the Roaring Twenties.

## "MODERN" DANCE

The decade called the Roaring Twenties has become associated with flappers, the Charleston, speakeasies, and

Prohibition. Between 1920 and 1929, the wealth of the United States as a nation doubled and, for the first time in history, more people were living in cities than on farms. These facts and festivities have tended to be the focus of historical accounts, even though the decade also brought conflict and devastation; the 1921 **Tulsa Race Massacre** was a horrific example of racialized violence, and some of the phenomenal artists associated with the Harlem Renaissance, including Josephine Baker, ended up pursuing careers in Europe rather than live in segregated settings in the United States. The Immigration Act of 1924 was another barrier to equity: as numbers of immigrants to the United States increased following World War I, policies were put into place to limit immigrants. These restrictions were driven by both concerns about job scarcity and ethnic prejudice:

> The Emergency Quota Act of 1921 established the nation's first numerical limits on the number of immigrants who could enter the United States. The Immigration Act of 1924, also known as the National Origins Act, made the quotas stricter and permanent. These country-by-country limits were specifically designed to keep out 'undesirable' ethnic groups and maintain America's character as a nation of northern and western European stock.[6]

The Immigration Act of 1924 completely excluded immigrants from Asia, thereby extending the Chinese Exclusion Act, formally Immigration Act of 1882, a U.S. federal law that was the first and only major federal legislation to explicitly suspend immigration for a specific nationality.[7] Restrictions on immigration remained in place for four decades, shifting only when the Immigration Act of 1965 changed America's ethnicity-based quotas and introduced a more ethnically neutral way of controlling immigration.[8] How did these policies impact dancers and dance history?

Within this environment of racialized exclusion during the 1920s, as Americans sought to define who they were and what they valued, the first full-time dance critics were appointed to positions in the United States and the first university degree in Dance was created at the University of Wisconsin-Madison. These educators and writers wielded tremendous influence on what constituted dance as an art form and as a subject of study, in the United States and abroad. John Martin, dance critic at the *New York Times* from 1927 to 1962, literally named and defined modern dance and its exemplars, describing Martha Graham as "the symbol of the modern dance."[9] Martin, who had been a theater administrator and playwright prior to becoming a dance critic, based his evaluation of great choreographers on their ability to communicate through kinesthesia, meaning the sensations we feel when we watch someone dancing. This criteria meant that he valued a stripped down aesthetic, without ornamentation or frivolous decoration, that communicated directly and intensely. Martin was not immune to the racism and xenophobia of this decade, and he contributed to a racialized discourse wherein white artists like Graham were elevated as innovative while Black dancers, such as Katherine Dunham, were viewed as "Negro" artists.

Margaret H'Doubler, the educator who developed the first degree in Dance, created a course of study that strategically separated her definition of dance from dancing created by communities of color. Although they differed in their definitions of dancing as a product and performance (John Martin) or a process for analyzing movement (Margaret H'Doubler), Martin and H'Doubler generated the terms and aesthetic hierarchies that critics and educators would use for decades in their evaluation of artistic work. Important to this analysis, their criteria emerged in the 1920s and 1930s, in between World Wars I and II, and would become entwined with ideologies of America as a nation, seen most vividly in Martha Graham's performance *Appalachian Spring*.

## MARTHA GRAHAM'S MODERN AMERICA

The notion of an ambiguous figure, meaning an image that presents double and at times conflicting messages, is an apt description of Martha Graham's *Appalachian Spring*. At first glance, this is a performance that depicts a loving and poignant story about a man and woman living on a frontier. It includes eight characters: at its premiere in 1944 they were the Husbandman (Erick Hawkins), the Bride (Martha Graham), the Pioneer Woman (May O'Donnell), the Preacher (Merce Cunningham), and four Worshippers (Nina Fonaroff, Pearl Lang, Marjorie Mazia, Yuriko).[10]

Each of the main characters presents their own movement qualities, which are tethered to their personality traits: the Husbandman constantly looks and reaches outward, while the Bride draws him in. The Bride's movement is as meticulous and worried as his is expansive and horizontally stretched. The Pioneer Woman is a solitary individual, uninvolved in the other characters' interactions and often dancing with a sense of duality: rooted in the ground, yet directing her extremities towards the sky. The Preacher contrasts with the Pioneer Woman's serenity: his dancing is boisterous and buoyant, and his jumps suggest exclamations made during a

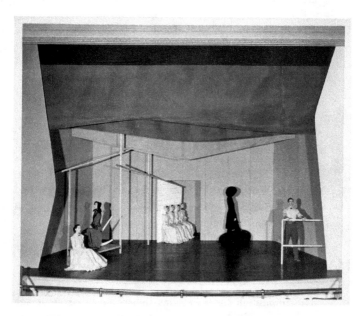

**Figure 5.2:** Photo of the 1944 performance of *Appalachian Spring*
Source: Elizabeth Sprague Coolidge Foundation Collection, Music Division, Library of Congress.

sermon. Graham's choreography emphasizes a sense of rugged individualism, an ideology tied to an American ethos, as each character dances independently, differently, and rarely in unison, except for the four Worshippers who often move together to convey devotion and conformity.

There is no hierarchal treatment of stage design, meaning no prominence given to center stage; instead, each character occupies a kind of home base, where they spend their time when they are not dancing, and all of the cast is on the stage throughout the 31-minute performance [see Figure 5.2].

This spacing generates a sense of democracy: it is egalitarian and anti-hierarchical, traits that politicians frequently referenced at this time. The performance evokes a sense of frugality that President Franklin D. Roosevelt shared during his 1937 Inaugural Address, "The test of our progress is not whether we add more to the abundance of those who have much; it is whether we provide enough for those who have too little." In a similar manner, the score by Aaron Copland, with its references to the Shaker tune "Simple Gifts," conveys directness and prudence, also traits that Americans sought to embody, especially after the Great Depression. The set design by Isamu Noguchi, with its stark references to a fence – a symbol of claiming territory – and a domestic interior conveyed through a fragile slice of a house, encapsulates the sparseness of this landscape, unadorned and unornamented. Each of these elements – choreography, music, and set design – contribute to the elevation of certain definitions of American life and modern dance. These definitions reinforced one another at a time when the country was actively defining itself in opposition to other identities and cultures.

In 1930, Graham stated in an essay called "Seeking an American Art of the Dance" that choreographers cannot imitate dances of other nations, and the "dance form of America" must "differ greatly from that of any other country."[11] Graham explains,

> the Oriental dance, least comprehensible of all, with its hieratic symbolic gesture, impossible of assimila-

tion because of its involved philosophy—and last the German dance, nearest to us of all, dangerously near, the voice of a determined, tired, but forever mentally undefeated people.[12]

Here we see Graham, a white woman, associating herself – and "us" – with German people, and othering Asian and Asian-American communities. Graham's essay continues, identifying "two primitive sources" of this essentially American dance form, "the Indian and the Negro."[13] In early drafts of her synopsis for *Appalachian Spring*, Graham initially included a character named the "Indian Girl." As scholar Jacqueline Shea Murphy notes, the first and second versions of the script for the piece include this "Indian Girl" as a major character.[14] By the time the performance had its premiere at the Library of Congress in 1944, this character had disappeared, and the production, in both form and narrative, presented Graham's vision of whitewashed American life and American dance. She emphasized this racialized view in her 1930 essay about American Art: "It is life as seen through our eyes and manifested in our art that is essential and of value to the future of dance."[15]

*Appalachian Spring* continues to hold tremendous appeal, most notably as an exemplar of modern dance. Writing in June of 2020, Melissa Strong states, "*Appalachian Spring* captures the essence of modern dance, as well as modernism itself, in drawing from the traditions of the past, breaking with them, and forging something **interdisciplinary** and new."[16] So far in this analysis I have attended to what is foregrounded in this collaboration between Graham, composer Copland, and designer Noguchi. By shifting our lens and bringing the background into focus, we can see how modern dance both shaped, and was shaped by, global conflicts. Graham wrote to Copland about *Appalachian Spring*, noting that she wanted to evoke "something nostalgic in the lyrical way and yet completely unsentimental and strong."[17] Nostalgia means a sentimental longing for the past and is often a fabricated or skewed version of what has actually occurred. *Appalachian Spring* relies on an imagined past that depicts frontier life with no strife, no conflict, no hunger, no genocide, and no hardship. In 1943, when Graham began working on the performance, the United States had already established internment camps for people of Japanese ancestry, authorized through President Franklin Roosevelt's Executive Order 9066.[18] On the West Coast in 1942, roughly 120,000 people of Japanese ancestry, two-thirds of them United States citizens, were forcibly relocated and incarcerated, usually in bleak camps throughout the Rockies and Southwest. They were not charged with any crime, and the vast majority were loyal Americans.[19]

The white American backlash against Japanese Americans in the United States had a dramatic personal effect on Noguchi, motivating him to become a political activist. In 1942, he cofounded Nisei [second-generation Japanese American] Writers and Artists Mobilization for Democracy, a group dedicated to raising awareness of the patriotism of Japanese Americans, and voluntarily entered the Poston War Relocation Center in Arizona where he remained for six months.[20] *New Yorker* columnist Kathleen Massara notes:

> His hope was to start an arts-and-crafts program, which could be replicated in the other camps. Such a program, he thought, would not only provide training opportunities for internees but make life more bearable in the desert. He also had a plan for a park and recreation area, and an adobe columbarium, chapel, and crematorium inspired by the work of his friend Buckminster Fuller.[21]

Instead of building this program, he was held captive in the camp, and Noguchi wrote an essay that he sent to *Reader's Digest* (never published), that included the insight, "I begin to see the peculiar tragedy of the Nisei as that of a generation of transition accepted neither by the Japanese nor by America. A middle people with no middle ground."

What happens when Noguchi's experiences of internment become the figure instead of the background in images of *Appalachian Spring*? Instead of a production that presents one image of a patriotic and nationalistic America, we also notice how these concepts of home and belonging are reserved for white and privileged Americans. *Appalachian Spring* presents a propagandistic message that elevates opportunities and access for a select few, while ignoring the hardship and injustices experienced by so many others. Juxtaposing images of Noguchi's fence in the performance with photos from internment camps by Toyo Miyatake throws into sharp relief the ambiguity of these images. Whose story is being told through Graham's choreography, and whose story is being rendered invisible? At times, the archival material of dance history, like these images of *Appalachian Spring*, is most valuable when examined for what it obscures, as well as what it foregrounds.

This analysis brings into focus how performances not only reflect cultural values and ideologies, but also impose and enforce certain worldviews. It is also important to note that one performance cannot represent all of the work called modern dance created between World Wars I and II: labels always impose a false sense of unity among choreographic works that often differ in their creative processes and intent. Nevertheless, analyzing *Appalachian Spring* as a performance that reveals the tensions between figure and ground, or what is presented and what is occluded, offers a framework for better understanding how categorization is contingent. Choreographers like Graham were not operating in a vacuum; they were part of networks of support that included critics, audiences, patrons, dancers, and artistic collaborators. Merce Cunningham, a performer with Graham's company from 1939 to 1945, is the focus of the next section on postmodern dance, and another exemplar of an ambiguous figure; an artist who has been historicized as a radical innovator, yet whose performances reveal an indebtedness to other cultures and worldviews.

## POSTMODERN DANCE AND MERCE CUNNINGHAM

At first glance, Graham's *Appalachian Spring* and Cunningham's *RainForest* present stark contrasts: in *RainForest*, there is no narrative, and no "characters" like the Bride or Husbandman.

Instead, there is a cast of seven dancers wearing flesh-colored leotards and tights that have been ripped so as to appear rough and unpolished. Silver, rectangular balloons float around the space. There is no apparent connection between steps and musical score, but rather Cunningham has choreographed the steps without any music and the dancers first hear the score by David Tudor when they perform *RainForest* for the first time, on March 9, 1968, at Buffalo State College.

Yet there are consistencies and commonalities found in work by Graham and Cunningham: both rely on a single white choreographer as the "creator" of a performance that is then performed by studio-trained dancers who are predominantly white. The training that these dancers pursue is steeped in codified techniques that cater to particular body types and canonical notions of flexibility, strength, and physical virtuosity. This is not dancing that anyone or everyone could participate in, and this exclusivity is part and parcel of the segregation of these white dance techniques named for their creators from dancing that is collectively created and nurtured. The atmosphere created by dancers in *RainForest* is one of exploration and indeterminacy. There are no struggles or conflicts; dancers interact like forest creatures greeting one another in a playful repartee.

An evocative moment features a male-identifying dancer standing behind a female-identifying dancer who is seated with her knees bent, her back against his shins. They are both reaching their arms and circling their wrists, their hands held like fists, as if their arms are tendrils emerging from the earth. He bends down, placing his hands around her armpits to lift her and she extends her body and twists. He holds her for a moment, her feet still on the floor, and they both look to see what's behind them: balloons, another dancer standing still, his back to the audience. Then she is gently returned to her seated position, and the tendril explorations begin again. Other sections feature fantastic balances and quick, darting phrases that scatter the balloons.

Watching *RainForest*, I feel as if I am peering into a space-age terrarium, where the reptiles are replaced by humans, and there is no longer any flora. There is an **Apollonian** quality that emphasizes exquisite shapes and lines, and almost no eye contact or emotional expression. By not imposing a narrative on this scene, and not forcing connections among the movement, music, set, or costumes, Cunningham relinquishes much of the control that modern choreographers coveted. Allowing audiences to make their own connections between his choreography, Tudor's score, and Andy Warhol's balloons could be interpreted as a response to the authoritarian governments that dominated World War II in Germany, Italy, and Japan. Instead of a choreographer who dictates what collaborators should make, or even what steps should follow one another, Cunningham embraced chance procedures, and drew inspiration from the *I-Ching*, a classic Chinese text. But his process was not a wholly democratic enterprise.

The background of the 1960s contrasts starkly with the randomness, disconnection, and sparseness of Cunningham's aesthetics: numerous uprisings and demonstrations, throughout the world, including anti-war and civil rights protests, rocked countries and cities. In January 1968, months before the premiere of *RainForest*, the U.S. and South Vietnamese militaries sustained heavy losses as a result of the Tet Offensive, orchestrated by Ho Chi Minh and leaders in Hanoi. In the United States, athletes, artists, and politicians broke color barriers in varied sectors, and these breakthroughs happened alongside tragic events: Malcolm X was assassinated in 1965, and Martin Luther King Jr. in 1968. While Cunningham is often regarded as a radical innovator, there were other artists, notably Black artists, who were forging new forms of expression, quelling violence, and assuaging grief and sorrow.

On April 5, 1968, the day after Dr King's assassination, Black Americans rioted in 110 cities, and James Brown was due to perform in Boston, Massachusetts. Mayor Kevin White and Brown decided to proceed with the show and televise it since they realized people could not resist watching a James Brown concert. Their plan worked: thousands of viewers watched the televised concert and the streets of Boston were quieter than usual. In spite of this widespread appeal and socio-political impact, James Brown is rarely considered alongside the postmodern dancers and choreographers in dance history textbooks, including the often-circulated *Terpsichore in Sneakers* by Sally Banes.

One scholar who does analyze the political and artistic significance of Black artists is Cornel West, and his writing foregrounds the figures who have been relegated to the "background" in dance history. West describes Black dancers, historically and currently, generating a "kinetic orality," a type of speaking through movement that resonates with a "combative spirituality," a sense of "historical patience, subversive joy, and daily perseverance in an apparently hopeless and meaningless historical situation."[22] Offering examples of this combative spirituality, West cites Muhammad Ali's footwork, James Brown's dancing, and a Martin Luther King Jr. sermon. Placing these performances alongside white artists like Cunningham, who is frequently noted for his postmodern tendencies, the contours of the figure and background become vivid. Postmodern dance, as defined by white critics and historians, is a realm for predominantly white artists. West calls attention to this exclusivity:

> For too long, the postmodernism debate has remained inscribed within narrow disciplinary boundaries, insulated artistic practices, and vague formulations of men and women of letters. The time has come for this debate to be moved more forthrightly into social theory and historiography. To do so is to raise methodological questions about historical periodization, demarcation of cultural practices and archives, and issues of politics and ideology.[23]

While Cunningham and other white artists are lauded by white critics for being innovative and postmodern, what happens when we widen our lens and interrogate the borders between background and figure, to ask how and why Black artistry is not included?[24] Postmodern dancers celebrated by critics and historians include Steve Paxton, who was part of Cunningham's company and co-created his own approach to partnering with Nancy Stark Smith, called contact improvisation. In California, postmodern dancer Anna Halprin has been praised for introducing improvisation-based, site-specific, and therapeutic projects. Meanwhile, all of these characteristics are present in dancing of the Ohlone peoples, Native Americans who have made "site-specific" work for millennia in the Bay Area. While Cunningham's, Paxton's, and Halprin's projects and performances tend to be the figures that occupy prominent places in dance history; every analysis of dance categories is an opportunity to investigate disciplinary borders.

In the 1960s and 1970s, performer James Brown, dancer Cholly Atkins, and countless others provided kinesthetic and acoustic experiences that shaped protests and uprisings, made evident in songs like "Dancing in the Streets," the 1964 hit by Martha and the Vandellas. Mary Wilson of the Supremes remembers Atkins, who choreographed performances for Motown acts, as on a par with Fred Astaire, and notes it was "a shame he didn't receive all the recognition he deserved."[25] Atkins cultivated a Motown look that communicated sleekness, polish, precision, and effortless class. Leonard Pitts Jr., a Pulitzer Prize winning columnist, looked back on Atkins's career in 2003 and remembers watching his distinct choreography: "[I]f you were a black kid—heck, a white one, too—you gaped at what you saw. You wondered how they moved like that. How they came to 'be' like that."[26] Artists like Atkins and Brown ushered in new definitions of dance and performance, yet often remain backgrounded while postmodern artists like Cunningham, Halprin, and Paxton are recognized.

When you think of postmodern dance, what is most prominent? Who is the figure and what is the background, and why? The tendency to overlook innovations by BIPOC artists changed in the wake of civil rights movements, especially when soldiers returned to the United States after fighting in the Vietnam War, and demanded better treatment and rights. Alongside uprisings for women's rights, rights of Indigenous nations, and African-American rights, new dance companies were established that furthered these agendas: in 1980

Daystar (Rosalie Jones) established the first dance company in the U.S. created with all-native performers and specializing in the portrayal of personal and tribal stories of Indian America; in 1982 Bill T. Jones/Arnie Zane Dance Company was established; in 1984, Urban Bush Women was founded by Jawole Willa Jo Zollar, who began her dance training with Joseph Stevenson, a student of Katherine Dunham, and traces her influences to icons like Cholly Atkins, Dianne McIntyre, and Daniel Nagrin.[27]

# CONTEMPORARY DANCE

Today, around the world, choreographers present performances that juxtapose individual and collective existences, and that provide insights into identities, cultures, and histories. Jack Gray, a Māori contemporary dancer, choreographer, teacher, facilitator, and writer, is the Artistic Director of Atamira Dance Company, a nationally-funded collective established in 2000 in Aotearoa.[28] Māori ancestors were the first people to settle in Aotearoa, with European settlers arriving about 400 years later, when Dutch explorers landed in 1642. In 1840 the Treaty of Waitangi was signed, marking an agreement between Governor William Hobson and 500 Māori chiefs, but the terms of the agreement were soon violated by European settlers. Similar to histories of conquest and colonization that created the United States, the history of Aotearoa includes land confiscations, incarcerations of Indigenous peoples, and genocide. Currently, Māori are the country's largest minority, and include 16.7% of the population. Through his artistic practices, Jack Gray cultivates Indigenous approaches towards enhanced relationships among place, people, and potential.

During an interview held in 2021 on Waitangi Day, Gray spoke about the tensions between internal and external narratives, and the ways he has navigated these as an artist:

> I always find it interesting when we chat up against what our internal dialogue is wanting to say, as opposed to how the outside experience is manifesting... [T]

here are these ever-present navigations [involving] our personal image, ourselves, our body, our reality, our memories, our familial histories, our cultural histories and our present. I guess all of those things create the day that we come into... Empires come and go and collapse as easily as they are oppressive and stamp their mark. And yet yes, their emperor lives on, their traces filter through. And I guess, we can't shut things out. It's better to work with those currents.[29]

Working with currents, nurturing connections, and emphasizing interdependence are themes that run throughout Atamira Dance Company's projects and history, and are also apparent in Gray's career. Against notions of art-making as dictating or commanding one perspective or narrative, Atamira amplifies contemporary Māori culture and artistic philosophies, and draws on personal stories, lineages, and *whakapapa*, a Māori word that translates to "a place in layers," meaning ancestral land, genealogy, and context or belonging. Unlike performances that set up a transactional encounter with "watchers" and "performers," Gray says, "[T]here are no givers and receivers... the gathering space that we're making together is a negotiation that finds its way through patience and a willingness to sometimes string moments together that may not immediately bring about a clear understanding."[30] More specifically, about his role as a director, Gray notes, "I don't know who's going to come and why they're going to be challenged, confronted and transformed because that's not my job to do. My job is to create spaces that evoke the energy to do so."[31]

If an ambiguous figure blurs borders between background and figure, Atamira Dance Company brings this approach into performance itself, generating environments that encourage more malleable and dynamic relationships among dancers and audiences than was present in the earlier examples of modern and postmodern dance. Another crucial element in Atamira's creative process is the inclusion of dancers' heritage and lineages in the creation of performances. One example is *Memoirs of Active Service*, choreographed by Maaka Pepene, first performed in 2005, and restaged in 2009. It is based on the diaries of Pepene's grandfather, Charles John Murphy, who served during World War II, and also draws from Pepene's own experience with the Royal New Zealand Infantry Regiment. During this interdisciplinary production, video designed by Louise Potiki Bryant shows pages from the grandfather's diary, and the sound-score designed by Paddy Free includes songs and radio announcements from the 1940s. Pepene performed the role of his grandfather, and the role of the grandfather's wife was danced by Pepene's wife, Justine Pepene-Hohaia. Rather than dancers performing "characters," this production emphasized familial and cultural connections. In Gray's words, these relationships are vital to Atamira: "All the dancers require individual and personal connection to their role that creates the movement."

*Memoirs of Active Service* ended with the poignant last words, "Kamaumahara tonu tatou ki a ratou," which means, "We will remember them." Gray recalls a recent moment when he became choked up at the end of a rehearsal:

> I was just thinking about sacrifices made so that we can live in the world that we're living in today and this sort of the bravery is showing and then the resilience shown by the people who stay behind. And we call it a tangi. So tangi is a funeral, but it's also just crying... The tangi is a kind of energy and it's a vibration. So it's almost like I just shifted vibration.[32]

Reviews of *Memoirs* note its ability to activate emotional memories, associations with veterans, and admiration for loved ones who dedicate their lives to their country. The production honors the famous 28th (Māori) Battalion, one of New Zealand's most formidable fighting forces, and the score by Paddy Free incorporates the Māori Battalion Marching Song. This battalion included 20% of the 16,000 Māori in New Zealand who registered for service and served with distinction both at home and abroad during World War II. One dance critic wrote about *Memoirs of Active Service*, noting that "The violence of war, while a powerful presence, is overshadowed by the bonding between the men."[33]

Here again we see a multiplicity of perspectives amplified and uplifted, rather than one image or one narrative dominating the production.

Throughout our interview, Gray notes the insufficiencies of English to explain a concept and often uses Māori vocabulary to make a point comprehensible to an outsider. One example is the Māori word *mana*, which Gray translates as a

> non-religious spiritual power... [I]t's also about integrity and balance. And so other people can trample your mana by disrespecting you by not recognizing your resources by not believing what you're saying is yours, by denying your mana, the existence of your mana.

Projects initiated by Atamira cultivate *mana* and give *mana* to others. As the director of Atamira, Gray explains that a priority within his research and creative process is "thinking about values like, what are the common values to humankind?" Atamira's performances acknowledge and affirm a multiplicity of perspectives and connections among audiences and dancers. This approach contrasts with American modern and postmodern dance, which became genres associated with white artists and racialized histories of dance. Gray says about Atamira, "We are a collective, and the act of making dance is always together." This intention is inextricable from a Māori concept called *tuākana/teina*. Gray explains,

> A tuākana is an eldest sibling and the responsibility of the tuākana is always to teach the teina, the youngest sibling, always, it doesn't matter the age. And it's adopted in Maori schools. And so the kids who are a year older or something, they always have to turn it around and teach the kids how to do things... And I've been navigating that within the dance company in a way that's not hierarchical, but a way that is I guess embedded in sort of a gentle remembering of what it was like for each person to go through the parts where they were uncertain or unsure or unclear... And the secret really is that the teina also teaches the tuākana... Again, it connects what we call tikanga; tikanga is protocol. And

there are protocols of New Zealand society, and then there's just tikanga Māori, which is just a Māori thing that you would do.[34]

These principles of reciprocity and protocol are guiding perspectives of Māori and many other Indigenous cultures, and present a stark contrast to notions of domination, nostalgia, and individualism, which have been reproduced in American modern and postmodern dance.

Placing Gray's work as the figure against a background of other genres of dance, we notice its challenge to definitions of dance that uphold white supremacy and settler colonialism, and its radical assertion of Māori values and philosophies that are vital to global wellbeing. Placing *Memoirs of Active Service* in the foreground of Aotearoa dance, we notice the differences and contours created by contemporary performance as a genre: prior to the 1980s and 1990s, dance in institutional settings, such as universities and concert venues in Aotearoa, was dominated by modern dance and dance education from the United States. Margaret Barr, an American who had worked with Martha Graham, arrived in Auckland in 1940, and became an influential teacher and choreographer, working with students at the Auckland Theatre School at University College. It is fascinating to consider differences between Graham's *Appalachian Spring*, a nostalgic and propagandistic performance created during World War II, and Atamira's *Memoirs*. Graham's production brackets an image of Americana, drawing from Shaker music and notions of "rugged individualism," to present an idealized vision. *Memoirs of Active Service* connects audiences and performers through a shared experience of patriotic service and conflict, and highlights the vital contributions of Māori peoples to the country's history.

# CONCLUSION

Each of the productions analyzed in this chapter highlight relationships between global conflicts and choreography and provide ways of noticing how artists navigate personal, nationalistic, and political affiliations. The concept of an ambiguous figure, an image that can be interpreted in two very different ways, becomes a useful way of recognizing which perspectives are highlighted or foregrounded in these performances, and which are obscured. As an audience member I am enthralled by performances that can be interpreted and valued by different people, and in my research and teaching I encourage us to notice when one dance critic's or one historian's view comes to represent this multiplicity of perspectives. More specifically, I analyze how a writer's positionality influences the values and criteria brought to performances and the danger of a single story or a narrative that erases other perspectives.[35] While Martha Graham's production of *Appalachian Spring* may be praised as exemplifying modern dance, we can also interpret its narrative and design as exclusionary and idealized. Merce Cunningham may continue to be written about as a radical postmodern artist, yet we can also widen our lens on the 1960s and 1970s and acknowledge other radical innovators often omitted from dance history books, like Cholly Atkins and James Brown. Jack Gray and Atamira Dance Company make contemporary performances that amplify Indigenous perspectives and help us rethink our relationships to history, to dance, and to one another.

## FURTHER READING

Chatterjea, Ananya. *Heat and Alterity in Contemporary Dance.* Palgrave Macmillan, 2020. Chatterjea exposes the systemic exclusions embedded in the construction of categories like "contemporary dance" and analyzes the work of Germaine Acogny, Sardono Kusumo, Nora Chipaumire, Rulan Tangen, Lemi Ponifasio, Camille Brown, Prumsodun Ok, and Alice Sheppard.

Croft, Clare. *Dancers as Diplomats: American Choreography in Cultural Exchange.* Oxford: Oxford University Press, 2015. Croft describes touring programs created by the State Department of the United States and the networks of institutional support that promoted the work of certain choreographers and dance companies.

Dixon Gottschild, Brenda. *Digging the Africanist Presence in American Performance.* Westport: Greenwood Press, 1998. Dixon Gottschild highlights the tremendous influence of Africanist aesthetics on dance and choreography in the United States, and reveals how and why these influences are often undocumented or misattributed.

Hall, Stuart. "The West and the Rest: Discourse and Power," *The Formations of Modernity*. Cambridge: The Open University, 1992. Hall examines how discourses, such as "the West" or "Western civilization," are produced and maintained to assert power and to delimit which people and cultures have access to that power, as well as which do not.

Ross, Janice. *Moving Lessons: Margaret H'Doubler and the Beginning of Dance in American Education*. Madison: University of Wisconsin Press, 2000. Ross traces the development of the first dance degree program in the United States, created by Margaret H'Doubler at the University of Wisconsin-Madison.

Shea Murphy, Jacqueline. *The People Have Never Stopped Dancing: Native American Modern Dance Histories*. Minneapolis: University of Minnesota Press 2007. Shea Murphy provides both a historical and theoretical account of the importance of Native dance and amplifies the importance of dance's transformative abilities.

Wong, Yutian. *Choreographing Asian America*. Middleton: Wesleyan University Press, 2010. Wong analyzes relationships between Asian America and American dance history, paying close attention to the intertwining of representations, identities, and stereotypes.

# TIMELINE

1200s – Māori ancestors settle in Aotearoa.

1642 – Dutch explorers land in Aotearoa.

1915 – Edgar John Rubin conceptualizes Rubin's Vase.

1921 – Tulsa Race Massacre: a violent white mob kills hundreds of people and destroys the Greenwood District, also known as America's Black Wall Street.

1924 – The Immigration Act of 1924 limits the number of allowed immigrants to the United States.

1944 – *Appalachian Spring* is performed.

1965 – Malcolm X is assassinated.

1968 – The Tet Offensive, orchestrated by Ho Chi Minh and leaders in Hanoi, is launched in Vietnam.

1968 – Martin Luther King Jr. is assassinated.

1968 – Merce Cunningham creates *RainForest*.

2006 – *Memoirs of Active Service* is choreographed.

# BIBLIOGRAPHY

Adichie, Chimamanda. "Danger of a Single Story," *TED Global* July 2009. www.ted.com/talks/chimamanda_ngozi_adichie_the_danger_of_a_single_story?language=en (accessed March 15, 2021).

Channing, Carol and Terry Monaghan. "Obituary: Cholly Atkins," *The Guardian*, April 28, 2003. www.theguardian.com/news/2003/apr/29/guardianobituaries.artsobituaries (accessed March 15, 2021).

Dent, Michelle and MJ Thompson. "Bill T. Jones: Moving, Writing, Speaking," *TDR* Vol. 49, No. 2 (Summer 2005), 53.

Graham, Martha. *Blood Memory*. New York: Doubleday, 1991.

Graham, Martha. "Seeking an American Art of the Dance," in *Revolt in the Arts: A Survey of the Creation, Distribution and Appreciation of Art in America*, ed. Oliver M. Sayler. New York: Brentano's, 1930.

Hobsbawm, E.J. *Nations and Nationalism Since 1780*. New York: Cambridge University Press, 1990; reprint, 2008.

"The Immigration Act of 1924." *Office of the Historian*. https://history.state.gov/milestones/1921-1936/immigration-act (accessed March 15, 2021).

Martin, John. *The Dance*. New York: Tudor Publishing Company, 1946.

Massara, Kathleen. "The Japanese-American artist who went to the Camps to Help," *New Yorker* January 31, 2017. www.newyorker.com/culture/culture-desk/the-japanese-american-artist-who-went-to-the-camps-to-help (accessed March 9, 2021).

Pind, Jörgen L. "Looking back: Figure and ground at 100," *The British Psychological Society: The Psychologist* 25 January 2012, 90–91. https://thepsychologist.bps.org.uk/volume-25/edition-1/looking-back-figure-and-ground-100_(accessed March 15, 2021).

Pitts, Leonard, Jr. "Cholly Atkins Taught Stars." *Sun Journal*. May 3, 2003. www.sunjournal.com/2003/05/03/cholly-atkins-taught-stars/ (accessed March 15, 2021).

Shea Murphy, Jacqueline. *The People Have Never Stopped Dancing*. Minneapolis: University of Minnesota Press, 2007.

Thomas, Evan. "'Infamy' and 'The Train to Crystal City'." *New York Times*. April 21, 2015. https://www.nytimes.com/2015/04/26/books/review/infamy-and-the-train-to-crystal-city.html (accessed March 9, 2021).

West, Cornel. "Black Culture and Postmodernism," *Remaking History*. New York: The New Press, 1989.

Zollar, Jawole Willa Jo. "Listen, Our History is Shouting at Us: A choreographer confronts racism in dance," *Looking Out: Perspectives on Dance and Criticism in a Multicultural World*. New York: Schirmer Books, 1995.

# NOTES

1　Jörgen L. Pind, "Looking back: Figure and ground at 100," *The British Psychological Society: The Psychologist* 25 (January 2012), 90–91. Accessed March 15, 2021: https://thepsychologist. bps.org.uk/volume-25/edition-1/looking-back-figure-and-ground-100

2　E.J. Hobsbawm, *Nations and Nationalism Since 1780* (New York: Cambridge University Press, 1990; reprint, 2008). Hobsbawm argues that nationalism encompasses "needs, longings and interests of ordinary people." (10).

3　Examples of these history books include *No fixed points: Dance in the 20th Century* by Nancy Reynolds and Malcolm McCormick; *Ballet and Modern Dance* by Susan Au and James Rutter; *Ballet and Modern Dance: a concise history* by Jack Anderson; *The Dance* by John Martin; *Dance: A Short History of Classic Theatrical Dancing* by Lincoln Kirstein

4　Michelle Dent and MJ Thompson, "Bill T. Jones: Moving, Writing, Speaking," *TDR* Vol. 49, No. 2 (Summer 2005), 53.

5　This is the Māori word for New Zealand.

6　"Closing the Door in Immigration," *National Park Service*, July 18, 2017. Accessed March 15, 2021: www.nps.gov/articles/closing-the-door-on-immigration.htm

7　"The Immigration Act of 1924," *Office of the Historian*. Accessed March 15, 2021: https://history.state.gov/milestones/1921-1936/immigration-act

8　"The Immigration Act of 1924," *Office of the Historian*. Accessed March 15, 2021: https://history.state.gov/milestones/1921-1936/immigration-act

9　John Martin, *The Dance* (New York: Tudor Publishing Company, 1946), 131.

10　Recording available here: www.youtube.com/watch?v=-WUcLG49qYw

11　Martha Graham, "Seeking an American Art of the Dance," in *Revolt in the Arts: A Survey of the Creation, Distribution and Appreciation of Art in America*, ed. Oliver M. Sayler (New York: Brentano's, 1930), 252.

12　Graham, "Seeking," in Sayler's *Revolt in the Arts*, 250.

13　Ibid., 254–255.

14  Jacqueline Shea Murphy, *The People Have Never Stopped Dancing* (Minneapolis: University of Minnesota Press, 2007), 148.

15  Graham, "Seeking," in Sayler's *Revolt in the Arts*, 250.

16  Melissa Strong, "Modern Dance: then and now," *BroadStreetReview.com*, June 30, 2020. Accessed March 15, 2021: www.broadstreetreview.com/dance/a-1944-recording-of-martha-grahams-appalachian-spring-is-streaming-for-free#

17  Martha Graham, *Blood Memory* (New York: Doubleday, 1991), 228.

18  Executive Order 9066 is a harrowing example of the ways that the U.S. Government can eradicate human rights overnight: this order, issued by President Roosevelt, enabled the evacuation of all persons "deemed a threat to national security." For more information, visit: www.ourdocuments.gov/doc.php?flash=false&doc=74

19  Evan Thomas, "'Infamy' and 'The Train to Crystal City'," *New York Times* (April 21, 2015). Accessed March 9, 2021: www.nytimes.com/2015/04/26/books/review/infamy-and-the-train-to-crystal-city.html

20  Kathleen Massara, "The Japanese-American artist who went to the Camps to Help," *New Yorker* (January 31, 2017). Accessed March 9, 2021: www.newyorker.com/culture/culture-desk/the-japanese-american-artist-who-went-to-the-camps-to-help

21  Idem.

22  Cornel West, "Black Culture and Postmodernism," *Remaking History* (New York: The New Press, 1989), 93.

23  West, 88.

24  While Gus Solomons Jr. was a performer in *RainForest* and a member of Cunningham's company from 1965 to 1968, there were no Black women in Cunningham's company over the course of its 56 years (1953–2009). This became glaringly apparent in 2015 when the Stephen Petronio Company performed *RainForest* and Davalois Fearon was part of the cast. For more information, see the documentary *If The Dancer Dances* (2019).

25  Carol Channing and Terry Monaghan, "Obituary: Cholly Atkins" *The Guardian*, April 28, 2003. Accessed March 15, 2021: www.theguardian.com/news/2003/apr/29/guardianobituaries.artsobituaries

26  Leonard Pits, "Cholly Atkins Taught the Stars," *Sun Journal*, May 3, 2003. Accessed March 15, 2021: www.sunjournal.com/2003/05/03/cholly-atkins-taught-stars/

27  Jawole Willa Jo Zollar has written an article that describes how racism has influenced dance criticism, and by extension, dance history and disciplinary formations: "Listen, Our History is Shouting at Us: A choreographer confronts racism in dance," *Looking Out: Perspectives on Dance and Criticism in a Multicultural World*. New York: Schirmer Books, 1995.

28 This is the Māori word for New Zealand. For more information on Māori culture, visit: https://teara.govt.nz/en/biculturalism?utm_source=newzealandnow.govt.nz

29 Jack Gray, Interview with author, February 6, 2021.

30 Gray, Interview.

31 Gray, Interview.

32 Gray, Interview.

33 Gray, Interview.

34 Gray, Interview.

35 For more on the danger of a single story, please view Novelist Chimamanda Adichie's lecture: www.ted.com/talks/chimamanda_ngozi_adichie_the_danger_of_a_single_story?language=en

# CHAPTER 6

# Dance and Social Justice
## Retracing the Steps of Michio Itō

*Dana Tai Soon Burgess*

Both sides of my family came to America as refugees. My mother's family immigrated in 1903 from Seoul, Korea to Hawaii, then an American Territory. They were among the first wave of Koreans to escape political and religious persecution under a deteriorating monarchy as the Empire of Japan vied for control. On the island of Oahu, they worked for three generations on plantations picking sugar cane and pineapple. My Caucasian father's family immigrated in the 1800s from Germany and Ireland, to Albany, New York to escape famine.

My parents, both visual artists, met in the early 1950s at Cranbrook Academy of Art in Michigan. Lifelong love was forged there from their mutual passion for making art. They married and ultimately settled in Santa Fe, New Mexico and raised two children. Art – painting and weaving – was the language that bridged their East and West cultures. This home environment incubated and nourished in me the skills to navigate my bi-racial Asian American identity, as well as confidence in the validity of my own individuality. Early on, dance, unbound by the restraints of spoken and written word, had become my own art, a thrilling kinesthetic language to express my inner emotional terrain. Art and the natural ease of my parents' bi-racial love infused my every day. No doubt, my parents' powerful influences continue to guide me in my role today as the Smithsonian's first-ever Choreographer-in-Residence, appointed in 2016 and based at the National Portrait Gallery in Washington, D.C.

DOI: 10.4324/9781003185918-6

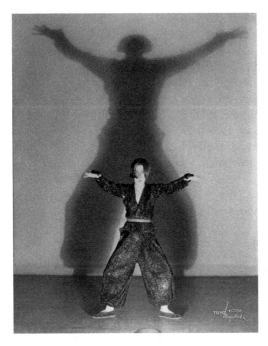

**Figure 6.1:** Michio Itō in *Pizzacati*, 1929. Photographer: Tōyō Miyatake.

Over the three decades of my professional career as a choreographer, I have dedicated myself to creating dances that animate the historic Asian American experience. Dance permits me to contextualize contemporary cultural realities for a wide audience.

In the midst of the current resurgence of organized as well as spontaneous individual anti-Asian attacks, I confront anew my own "otherness" in American society, the collisions as well as the rich confluence of my two cultures. How does the "other" – either the hyphenated being or the transplanted person of another race or country of origin – not suffer their own alienation, as a default status, ever on the outside, marginalized, excluded, tethered to America with a caveat, a qualifier deemed "less than?" Consider: the hyphenated brand, this permanent tattoo, is never invoked to signify "more than." Through movement I address the questions: how do we "others" resist and how do we adapt? And how does dance best serve as a story-telling medium, one that can inform, enlighten, and present potential understanding, empathy, and remedy?

"The medium *is* the message," as the late philosopher and seminal communication theorist Marshall McLuhan indelibly coined in 1964.[1] That is, the very form we use to communicate ideas plays a crucial role in determining the impact, the perceptions, intention, reception, and the meanings of the message one seeks to deliver. In that very same way, I see physical movement as Social Justice movement. In short, Movement itself as a Movement.

As an undergraduate in the dance program at the University of New Mexico I struggled to identify an Asian American modern dance lineage with which I might align. Then one day a dance history professor said, "Dana, you must learn about Michio Itō. He was a modern dance pioneer, now rarely talked about.... follow the trail of Itō." I wondered, why was Michio Itō (c.1893–1961) seemingly excluded from occupancy of his rightful place in American modern dance history? Dr. Judith Bennahum's words that day set me on a decades-long transformative journey back in time.

Through the investigation of Michio Itō's art and life, I learned about the whitewashing of history and the systemic amnesia, the hemorrhagic loss of Asian American stories. It led me to internalize and embody his repertory as a form of social justice and restoration. Itō's career points to the ramifications of shifting socio-political perspectives of the East between the two World Wars.

Born in Japan, Itō chose America as his home and built a prestigious career spanning from New York City to Los Angeles that included touring, teaching, and work on Broadway and in Hollywood. Early in his career, Itō was heralded as the "exotic other," but in 1941, less than three decades later, after building a successful school and dance company, he would be vilified as a symbol of the so-called "Yellow Peril" – a threat from the East.

With the attack on Pearl Harbor on December 7, 1941, his successes would be eclipsed by U.S. wartime policies. He was imprisoned soon after and repatriated to Japan in 1943. Itō's legacy in America has been almost forgotten. By resurrecting Itō's story and performing his dances, I have been able to open discussions with audiences about a period of American history that is so painful and shameful that it is often unspoken by either the victims or the government. Healing begins with disclosure.

I grew up in the 1970's in Santa Fe, New Mexico in a Hispanic neighborhood called *Casa Solana*, "house in the sunshine." My family was new to this established community, our physical appearances conspicuous as "others." Here, unbeknownst to me at that time, I would stand in the footprints of Michio Itō.

When I was nine years old, I often played "war" with my classmate David Gonzales in his front yard, whose boundaries were girded by a chain link fence. We ran, jumped, rolled, ducked, hid, and took cover from each other's pretend bullets, yelling, "Pow! I got you!" and "You're dead!" One day, his grandfather, who had been sitting on the porch, approached me and said, "*Chinito*," (Spanish for "little Chinese man") "with this metal fence around you, you remind me of the Japanese prisoners that used to be here during the war." I had no idea what he was referring to, but I shivered, stung to my core. His snicker at my ignorance was all the more chilling. He gave no further description of his memory. But I would not play with David again. His grandfather's words were bullets I could not dodge.

I asked my father, "What did David's grandfather mean?" Dad had been in the Navy during WWII and surely knew the man's reference. "Dad, how could being Asian lead to being put in prison?" I studied my father's stricken face and considered my angular cheeks and almond eyes, facial features so different than his. And I am Korean, not Japanese. Were Asian features alone a reason that a person could be put in prison? Choosing his own words carefully, Dad explained that during WWII, yes, a prison for Japanese

Americans stood on the land upon which our neighborhood was now built. "Were they robbers and murderers?" I asked. He answered, "No, they were here because the President didn't trust Japanese Americans back then...." My father tried to explain that the American President had the power to take away the rights of citizens if he suspected that they could be dangerous. "Dana, the President... well, he made a big mistake." I was inconsolable. Light-headed. Terrified; it could happen to me.

Many years later, I would learn that Dad was referring to Executive Order 9066 which went into effect on February 19, 1942, just over two months after the December 7th bombing attack on Pearl Harbor by the Japanese. President Franklin D. Roosevelt signed the order, paving the way for the unjust and unilateral rounding up, removal, and imprisonment of approximately 120,000 individuals of Japanese ancestry in the United States. Two-thirds were American citizens, the other third were of Japanese ancestry living in America, Canada, and Peru.[2]

Having grown up on land that had been a prison camp – where the President had sentenced people just because they looked like me – would cast an indelible shadow of fear over my childhood that I could be grabbed and imprisoned just for being who I was: Asian American.

Beneath the soil of Casa Solana were the shallow ruins of a former Japanese American men's prison camp that had continued to operate right up until 1946, fewer than 30 years before my family moved to the neighborhood. The camp imprisoned over 4,500 men, a number equal to one-fifth the population of Santa Fe at the time (a little over 20,000). Here in 1943 Michio Itō would be imprisoned.[3]

## FROM ARTIST TO ENEMY

Michio Itō was born in Tokyo, Japan in 1892 or 1893 (records are not clear). His mother was Kimiye Iijima and his father was the architect Tamekichi Itō who had briefly left Japan for a Western education at the University of Washington. His parents were familiar with America and Europe and ignited their son's interest in the development of an East and West aesthetic.

Itō planned to venture from Tokyo to Paris for music studies. But his background and interest in Japanese theater and dance led him to Germany in 1912, where innovative concepts were percolating about how music and movement could be merged. He was then about 19 or 20 years old. Itō was short, lithe, slight; a black bob of hair framed his chiseled features and ears. In Hellerau, Germany he trained in a branch of kinesthetics called "eurythmics" at the Émile Jacques-Dalcroze Institute. Here, Itō was the only Asian among 300 enrolled students: an anomaly, an "exotic Easterner."[4]

Dalcroze, a Swiss educator and composer had designed "eurythmics." Itō experimented with its application, performing in and soon choreographing productions that emphasized the facility of the performer to move on the specific beats of a musical score. The technique held the body to be a musical instrument, that dancing steps, gestures, and even nuances of movement ought to be done as the direct physical embodiment of musical scores. Eurythmics would be a driving force behind many forms of early modern dance because it gave movement a framework by which it could have a direct synergy with music. Exercises were improvisational experimentations to coalesce rhythm and musical structure through movement.[5]

But this revolutionary fresh institute would be short-lived, in large part due to the advent of WWI. In the summer of 1914, Émile Jaques-Dalcroze took a trip to Switzerland and never returned to Hellerau. When Japan declared war on Germany at the end of 1914, Itō left the school and moved to England.[6]

In London Itō secured an engagement at the Coliseum Theatre where his appearances were advertised as the harmonious hybrid of European and Japanese dances.[7] European tastes were focused on "Orientalist" art, fashion, and dance.

The public's fascination with the East had been spurred by a resurgence of interest in the vivid images of Japanese woodblock prints, *Ukiyo-e*, that had flourished in the 17th to the 19th centuries and which now influenced the works of Western painters including Edgar Degas, Vincent Van Gogh, and Mary Cassatt. In 1872, French art critic Philippe Burty would coin this Western obsession "Japonisme."[8] Itō's dancing fed their sharpened appetites and imaginations and arguably, too, their appropriations.

Performing opportunities in London salons soon followed; Itō's edgy work attracted the admiration of poets Ezra Pound and William Butler Yeats and other influential artists and literati.[9] They mentored the young modern dancer and in 1916, Itō collaborated with Yeats to produce *At The Hawk's Well*, a one-act "movement play" presented in a "pseudo-Noh" drama format. *Noh* is a Japanese form of highly stylized theater that dates back to the 14th century and often features tales of supernatural beings.[10] Itō danced the *Hawk*, guardian of a magic well that bestowed immortality to any who drank from its water; one of three actors/dancers ("movers") and three musicians. His costume, designed by illustrator Edward Dulac, featured wings and painted skull cap inspired by ancient Egyptian wall paintings of the god Horus, often depicted as half-man and half-hawk. A Japanese modern dancer in a quasi-ancient Egyptian guise – London audiences could not get enough.[11]

Wendy Perron, the current editor of *Dance Magazine*, assesses the importance of this performance:

> He (Itō) saw an affinity between the wholeness of a Noh play and the Dalcrozian integration of dance and music. It was a kind of full circle whereby Ito's interest in the West brought him to Europe, and it was Western poets whose interest in Asia brought him back to his Japanese roots.[12]

*At the Hawk's Well* was an artistic coup for both Yeats and Itō, but in 1916 England was paralyzed with the early quivers of WWI, and that precluded any sustained performance runs.

That same year, Itō received a financially compelling contract from Oliver Morosco, an eminent American theater producer; Itō would add a much sought after Far East exoticism to Morosco's Western brand. But when Itō arrived in Manhattan, he was instead to dance in a "musical sex comedy" about two mate-swapping couples, dancing in front of their two beds."[13] He quit the contract. But now at least Itō had a New York base and he would pivot and build a following.

In 1916, Itō created his signature solo, *Pizzacati*, a short (90 second duration) visually arresting shadow dance, which he would go on to perform by popular demand throughout his career. He set the dance to composer Léo Delibes's *Pizzacato* extracted from his full score for the ballet *Sylvia* (1876) originally choreographed by Louis Mérante.[14] Pizzacato refers to a score marking that directs the plucking of violin strings by the instrumentalists. Itō danced *Pizzacati* in front of a massive golden screen, the reflective surface for his shadow. With a theatrical floor lamp placed at his feet that were positioned in a wide second stance, an imposing 12-foot shadow was cast on the backdrop to accentuate his every hand flick, stabbing arm thrusts, and tracings. Itō's hair was coiffed in his signature black bob, his costume, bespoke from the latest modern synthetic fibers, silver threads sparkling throughout its crisscrossed kimono top and black harem pants. His Asian garb was cinched tightly at the waist with a red silk *obi* (a Japanese cummerbund).

*Pizzacati* is stationery; the dancer never moves from his rooted spot on stage. Arms, hands, torso, head, and intense facial expressions each accentuate the pinched notes through serial gestures that occur at waist or shoulder level and above the head. In a last grand arm flourish, the dance folds at the waist and is dramatically plunged into darkness just as the spotlight blacks out on the last note of Delibes's score. Live violin plucking was seamlessly married to martial arts-like slices and jabs. Up until this time, the score had always been associated with ballet steps and this hybrid was radically new.

Itō's solo dances for revue-style shows featured exaggerated costumes from Egypt, Persia, China, India, Spain, and

Argentina. For his idiosyncratic tango, he would wear a Spanish hat, cropped bolero, and tight high-waisted pants. To dance as if a Beijing opera singer, he would don an opulent red silk robe embroidered with gold dragons, platform boots, and an elaborate headpiece with long pheasant feathers and pom-poms.[15]

Chameleon Itō took on personas from around the globe, ranging from *Chinese Dance: A Fable* (1918), *Bull Fighter* (1921), *Song of India* (1921), *Javanese* (1928), and *Spanish Fan* (1929). He would unavoidably fall into Western clichés of "others." These dances were set with classical music by Western European composers including Pyotr Ilyich Tchaikovsky, Isaac Albéniz, and Frédéric Chopin. Yet Itō did not claim to have based these fabricated, hybrid dances on scholarly research or reality. Instead, in a 1917 interview of Itō in *The New York Tribune* by Harriette Underhill, *Michio Itow* – titled with the phonetic spelling of his name – he elucidates his artistic reasoning, a desire to unify – while Underhill's words highlight the physical otherness of Itō:

> 'So!' he said, as he placed one little brown fist in the palm of the other hand. 'You see this fist, and you would say: what is this fist made of? We would see only this Shadow and we would say: what does this Shadow mean? In my dancing it is my desire to bring together the East and the West. My dancing is not Japanese. It is not anything-only myself. It is a series of poses; I am a sculptor, for I work, and I work over each pose until it means what I would have it mean'.

Underhill's racial colorization and diminution of his hand, a "little brown fist," demonstrates that she viewed the subject as different from herself, that he was not Caucasian. As he gained fame, his image would be portrayed by publications in ways intended to further accentuate his otherness. In 1926 an illustration by Carl Link of Itō in full Beijing Opera regalia would be the February cover of *Dance Magazine*; in 1927 Ivin Landgon's *1915 portrait of Itō* as a Samurai in full warrior garb added drama to the pages of another trade magazine, *The Dance*. The caption: "Michio

Ito – The famous character dancer in the mood and costume of a Japanese warrior." The price for his fame was racial stereotyping. By the 1930s he had crossed over into commercial advertisement. In Germany, during 1934, draped in an exotic shawl, Itō's image would be printed on souvenir cards (akin to American baseball trading cards) tucked inside boxes of Eckstein cigarettes, as an "American famed dancer and teacher."[16] Yes, Itō was now famous.

Itō taught classes in a rented studio above Carnegie Hall on 57th Street and 7th Avenue, midtown Manhattan headquarters for a prodigious performance and choreographic career. Itō attracted students to his Dalcrozian approach, as well as his theatrical representations of world cultures. His technique included the traditional Japanese arm movements and body positions he had studied in Japan.[17] Many of his students would become famous leaders in modern dance including Martha Graham. At 29, Graham danced in Michio Itō's *The Garden of Kama* (1923), a work featured in the **Greenwich Village Follies**, a series that featured short dances inspired by images from the East.[18]

Another who gained her start through Itō was Pauline Koner who toured with Itō's six other company members in the 1928–1929 season and would go on to become an essential member of the José Limon company from 1946–1960.[19]

This 1928–1929 tour included performances in California, which led to an invitation from the city of Pasadena for him to relocate his studio and headquarters there. Although by now well known, Itō had not become a financial success; Pasadena's offer lured him in 1929 to uproot from New York City. With financial assistance from the city, he relocated and set up a school and began to create large-scale productions – "symphonic choreographies" – for the newly built Rose Bowl stadium.[20]

In September of 1929, Itō staged *The New World Symphony*, at the Pasadena Rose Bowl set to the famous "New World Symphony" by Antonin Dvorak. This "movement choir" of 200 dancers was accompanied by the full symphonic Queen's

Hall Orchestra. The seating capacity of 20,000 would accommodate the city's boastful and prescient celebration of the installation of "the largest sun arc ever constructed!"[21] A sun arc is a spotlight used in the making of motion pictures.

He closed the show by dancing *Pizzacati* in front of a 40 by 125 foot golden screen. Musical conductor for the event, Henry Wood, recounts the success of this solo, "The dance itself was extraordinary, with only the upper portion of the body, the arms and head serving as the medium of expression. Recalled to stage he performed the dance a second time…"[22]

In California he also restaged *At the Hawk's Well*. This time Itō cast a talented and avid young acolyte, Lester Horton, as the *Hawk*, the role he had himself originated in London. Horton would later become an American modern dance icon in the 1940's and 50's, as well as becoming in turn Alvin Ailey's mentor.[23] Itō's technique featured two sets of ten codified arm and hand movements, one set "masculine," the other "feminine." The formalized sequences followed distinct pathways as the arms extended above the head, downward to the waist, bent across the chest, and finally hands covered the face prior to reaching straight upwards again. The palms pushing through space were the primary initiators of the arm movements. These two sets of serial arm cycles were placed on top of spiraling torques of the torso and barefoot walking patterns. Each movement corresponded to a tempo, i.e., 4:4 or 3:4, sped up or slowed down.

Itō would expand his work into film as actor, director, and choreographer in *Madam Butterfly* (1933) and *Booloo* (1938), among others. As Fred Astaire and Gene Kelly danced ballet, jazz, and tap on mainstream films, Hollywood would continue to exploit and commercialize Itō's exotic appeal. In *Booloo*, he was cast as the bare-chested chieftain of a primitive tribe in the jungles of Malay.[24]

But as the 1930s came to a close, anti-Japanese sentiment in America grew in tandem with global tensions leading up to World War II, and doomed Itō's momentum. On December 8, 1941, just one day after the attack on Pearl Harbor, the U.S. government would arrest Michio Itō. His business and personal connections to prominent individuals in both Japan and America suggested to a jittery republic that he posed a potential espionage threat to America. He had in fact been under FBI surveillance for months prior to the December 7th attack.

Itō was among the first individuals of Japanese descent living in America to be stripped of his human rights. He was initially held for two months at the Missoula, Montana Alien Detention Center. Here he was tried in early February of 1942. The trial board stated, "The subject is an alien enemy" and "The Board recommends INTERNMENT." On February 19, 1942, President Franklin D. Roosevelt signed Executive Order 9066, that mandated the immediate rounding up and incarceration of approximately 120,000 individuals of Japanese ancestry, predominantly at the time living on the West Coast of the United States. Itō was moved between internment camps at Fort Sill in Oklahoma, in April 1942, and then to Camp Livingston in Louisiana.[25]

Between 1942 and 1945 the United States government opened ten specific Japanese American prisons camps (so-called "internment camps") in desolate parts of Arkansas, Wyoming, Utah, and other remote areas and further populated existing detention and internment camps with Japanese Americans. Itō's final internment in 1943 would occur at the men's Santa Fe Internment Camp. From here he was unjustly deported to Japan, never to return to the United States where he had built a singular career as tastemaker, impresario, and pedagogue.

The remains of this prison camp were beneath my childhood neighborhood.[26] Through this shared land connection, beneath my feet, I most certainly absorbed my own nutrients as a dancer, born to ensure that Itō's legacy – and his quest to join East to West – would not be forgotten.

## RECURRING SERENDIPITIES AND EMBODIMENT

In 1988, I was 19 and an undergraduate student in the Dance Program at the University of New Mexico. My dance history teacher, Dr Judith Chazin Bennahum, recognized that I was the only Asian American student in the program and that I was sorely in need of an Asian American mentor. As a class assignment, she suggested that I write a paper about Michio Itō. She was quite familiar with his work. Knowing his story would nourish my own dance journey, she said. I had never heard of him. And even more telling: I had never even considered that there actually was an Asian American modern dance pioneer.

Over the next weeks, in the library, I found images and descriptions of him and his dances in a book, *Michio Itō: The Dance and His Dances*, written by Helen Caldwell, one of Itō's former dancers. Before me were page after page of photographs of a face with Asian features and a dancing silhouette that resembled my own body. Photos of the Itō arm positions intrigued me and made me yearn to learn his dances. But just as the interconnections of his impact upon modern dance history were making sense, his story abruptly ended with a few cryptic statements including, "Following Pearl Harbor all Japanese were evacuated from the West Coast. After a brief internment Michio Itō returned to Japan on the *Gripsholm*."

I asked Professor Bennahum, "What happened to him and why did he leave America when he had such a successful career?" She answered: "the Japanese Internment." Could it be that his legacy had been wiped out as well, due to racialized politics? I researched the Japanese Internment and learned how the ripple effect of Executive Order 9066 affected every single Japanese American community. I learned of Itō's imprisonment at the Santa Fe prison camp as well: an identity, a name and a face, on the mass victimhood that even my father did not know about.

Amazingly, my relationship to Itō went even further than dance and my neighborhood in Santa Fe. In reading about Itō's relationship to Martha Graham, I learned that visual artist and designer Isamu Noguchi had been one of his closest friends. Starting in 1935, over a period of three decades, Noguchi designed 20 of Martha Graham's sets. Noguchi's designs provided abstract psychological forms and landscapes that supported the themes of her choreography that ranged from stories of Americana to Greek tragedies. These included set designs for her iconic *Frontier* (1935), *Appalachian Spring* (1944), and *Cave of the Heart* (1946).[27] Because both of my parents were prominent abstract artists with connections to other Asian artists of stature, as a child of eight or nine, I had actually dined with Noguchi on several occasions. Typically, he, my parents, and Noguchi's half-sister, Ailes Gilmour (who had danced for Martha Graham), would get together routinely to discuss art. Noguchi was then in his early seventies and his sister Ailes in her sixties.

I had been privy to their conversations about art and dance influences. Suddenly all those memories came into focus: Noguchi's complaints about "Martha," that she was not giving him enough time to design a set for her dancers the time to explore his fabrications. The diaspora of broken youthful memories now, in a rush, all made sense. Martha was in fact...Martha Graham! And Ailes's memories of dancing were in fact priceless time capsules from an incubator of nascent American modern dance itself, a profession in which I so longed to play a part. Here was the vector meeting of Asian American artists attached to Itō. I was thunderstruck: two of my parents' friends had been close friends with Itō! The great inventive master of my idiom had been circling me my whole life.

I concluded my college paper on Itō with prescient words: "Someday I hope to learn the Itō dance technique and to perform his solo *Pizzacati*."

At 20, I moved to Washington, D.C. to pursue a professional dance career. I danced for both modern and neo-classical companies. Like Itō, I was a young, slight Asian American dancer with black bobbed hair. Because of my anomalous looks, choreographers struggled to cast me in their Eurocentric repertoire. My Asian American identity and perspective were absent in the programming. These generic roles felt like camouflage – concealment of at least half of my ethnicity.

From deprivation came initiative. I began to choreograph
my own original work on a group of eight Asian American
dancer friends. By 1993 I had created a taut portfolio of
dances that explored our Asian American family histories
of immigration. They were set to electronic modern musical scores. I returned time and again to lingering questions
I had surrounding Michio Itō. How exactly had he choreographed? How had he trained and coached his dancers?
What skills might I learn through mastery of his repertoire?
What self-knowledge might I gain?

By age 26 a passion took hold within me that was as strong as
my passion for dance. I longed to reclaim the history of Asian
America in modern dance, a history that had been denied to
me. I needed to embody the work of Itō in order to ensure
that Asian Americans were not forgotten in the canon of
modern dance. I had to learn his technique and his dances
before I could continue my own choreographic journey.

To do so, in 1994, I engaged my friend HIRO, a Japanese
American visual artist and civil rights activist. HIRO had
recently designed a set for one of my dances. She came from
a prominent Japanese American family and had ties with
individuals who had been incarcerated during WWII.[28] She
connected me with two of Itō's former female dancers who
serendipitously were living in the Washington, D.C region.
Lily Arikawa Okura (1919–2005), a soloist from Itō's
California era, and Michiko Yoshimura Kitsmiller (1926–
2017), who had trained with, and danced for, Itō in Japan
after his repatriation. HIRO also connected me with Saturo
Shimazaki, a male Itō dancer living in New York City who
had trained in Japan with Ryuko Maki, a Japanese protégé
of Itō who managed his dance school in Japan.[29]

Under the tutelage of Shimazaki, then in his fifties, Kitsmiller,
then 69, and Okura, then 76, my eight-member company,
learned the signature Itō "masculine" and "feminine" arm gesture series. We exercised Itō's "one arm lead," in which one
arm lags behind the other and right and left arms move independently instead of in unison. Itō's choreography typically
includes this patterning, and it can be a challenge to internalize

because it is in contrast to many contemporary modern dance techniques that focus on moving the body as a whole.

After a month, we had reached technical proficiency and were ready to apply our new vernacular to several of Itō's signature solos including *Pizzacati* (1916), *Ave Maria* (1914) – a sublime slow motion solo he created at the Dalcroze Institute – and *Tone Poem I & II* (1928) – movement *haikus* with a martial arts flair and which portray struggles against injustice – and finally, a work for five dancers, *En Bateau* (1929). This dance consists of poses in profile view that appear almost two-dimensional at times. These flat postures are juxtaposed to running and skipping patterns, inspired by the ebb and flow of ocean waves. Each of these dances was short, one to six minutes in length, daunting in their precision. At rehearsals, when I hit "play" on the studio stereo system and Schubert's *Ave Maria* gently sounded, Kitsmiller would rise and begin to move through her solo, *Ave Maria*. She danced with otherworldly ease. Nearly 70, she appeared untouched by time.

I traveled to New York for weekly coaching sessions from Shimazaki over several months. When Shimazaki demonstrated *Pizzacati*, he attacked each movement with musical exactitude. He demanded perfection through constant repetition, until the solo became second nature, embedded in my bones, sinew, and muscle memory. These pedagogues did not work with us for money or fame. They worked with us in order to ensure that Michio Itō's legacy would endure to influence yet another generation of dancers.

At breaks, Okura and Kitsmiller shared personal stories about Itō. Okura said that he was a perfectionist who gave notes to each dancer even when there were more than 200 in the cast. Kitsmiller said that for her solo *Ave Maria*, Itō had coached her every movement, hand placement, and even facial expressions.

Itō's transnational philosophy – that modern dance could lead to mutual cultural understanding – a bridge between East and West – was in no dispute. The respect they showed Itō, decades after dancing for him, was unwavering. But it was hard to get past that veneration and into certain parts of Itō, the man. Those were precisely the corners that I craved to have them illuminate. Conversations always abruptly stopped when I broached the subject of his emotions, especially about his incarceration and repatriation. I asked them, "What happened to Itō during World War Two?" Silence. I was left to hypothesize: was this silence molded from deep cultural shame for what had been done to them during the war? Was it perhaps combined with the fear that the Itō legacy would be stained if they spoke of this? Or was this a place that was so painful, so profane for Itō, that they did not want to conjure and perpetuate his inconsolable sorrow? Okura would only say, *shikata ga nai*. HIRO would explain to me that this is a phrase used by Japanese Americans who had lived through the trespasses and travesties of EO9066, in order to shut down conversation, and to save face in the naming of an injustice, exclusion, and bigotry that was beyond their control. Their resolute silence and this Japanese phrase affirmed that literally unspeakable pain, one that even after 50 years, was still just below the surface... It was a surface that, for Itō, was literally underneath my childhood home.

It wasn't until after our second public performance of the Itō dances, at the Dance Place in Washington, D.C., in January, 1995, before an audience of 150 people, that during a post-performance question and answer session, the truth of Itō's feelings would be given words. HIRO asked about the impact of EO9066 on Itō. Shimazaki replied, "World War Two tore out his heart, and his life."[30] It had taken the physical reanimation of Itō's work and the convergence of his devotees to assemble in a theater, a place of public healing, to acknowledge the traumas and erasure that Itō had experienced. After his deportation, Itō never returned to the United States and although his career in Japan would continue, his eminence in the history of American modern dance – his literal footprints – were made to fade away.

Michio Itō died in Tokyo in 1961. I ponder, 60 years later, how modern dance would see Itō today if he had not been deported. Would dance students avidly study the Itō technique at studios and university dance programs across the country? Would his company and dance studio still thrive? Would students equally learn about the artistic importance of Michio Itō, as they do Martha Graham?

In our current national turbulence around race and "otherness," around nationalism – and who is and is not entitled to protections for their human and civil rights – I consider Itō's life and artistry anew. I see in *Pizzacati*'s towering shadow the intractable racialized politics that entangled Itō and eclipsed his American career. I believe his signature solo best encapsulates the metaphor of the negative societal and political pressures that continue to haunt the Asian body, the Asian experience in America.

Whenever I perform *Pizzacati*, I experience a feeling akin to entering battle. Stoked with the specificity of the Itō technique and hundreds of rehearsals, I feel like David preparing to fight Goliath. Prior to the moment of performance, coiffed as Itō with my black hair in a bob, cinched and costumed, I wait alone in the dark for the curtain to rise, the spotlight to illuminate, the music to begin. This potent anthemic work allows me to jab and punch, to present ferocity of focus and a determination and alacrity of body movements that defiantly rage against subjugation. The invisible enemy is no person. It is bigotry. The experience is cathartic, a rite that rids me of the stereotypes of the often effeminized, hypersexualized, objectified, and vilified Asian American body. I am no one's toy. I am not a thing.

*Pizzicati* was never "just a dance;" rather it was a confrontation with societal stereotypes, systemic racist policies, and micro and macro aggressions that had chipped away at my identity and pride. Here, I am able to dance choreography that represents how I look and feel, that portray me as strong and that was created by a like-minded artist who also shared my deep sense of "otherness." *Pizzacati* is a celebration of that very "otherness."

Itō's artistry has informed my belief that the reanimation of a choreographer's dances can be a journey of remembrance, resilience, and in the case of this work, one of effective protest. Here is the transformative process of mentorship through movement resuscitation. Learning the Itō technique and performing *Pizzacati* has led me to truly understand why Itō is barely mentioned in the canon of American modern dance. Our society has an inherent discomfort with acknowledging its through-line of **systemic racism**. Now, each time I reset *Pizzacati* on a young dancer, I consider it a platform through which to openly communicate the long and troubled history of Asian Americans. And Michio Itō dances thrillingly, once again.

Itō's journey is unfortunately not an anomaly in the arts, there are similar journeys in which politics have impacted the lives and work of artists not only in the field of dance, but also in the visual arts and even in Hollywood. Acclaimed Chinese sculptor and architect Ai Weiwei has created monumental works which have often included commentary on social injustices and political corruption in China. This has made him an ongoing political target. Ai Weiwei was arrested by the Chinese government in 2011 and held in secret detention for 81 days before pressure from the international community forced his release. He lives outside of China today. Film and television star Jane Fonda has also dealt with political backlash. Her anti-war stance during the Vietnam War, led to her being blacklisted in Hollywood in the 1970's and almost 50 years later she is still considered controversial for her anti-war stance.

To me, *Pizzacati* is the tangible representation – a portrait, painted in choreography – of the phantasm that America does not want to face, the erasing of Asian contributions to America – in all of its history texts and in its artistic programming. Systemic racism has touched every facet of our society. Repertory can be perceived as the passing of movement knowledge from one body to another, and that is one layer of the skin. More deeply, more profoundly, and viscerally, it is the naked sharing of embodied stories of struggle and pain. *Pizzacati* has become a reveille, a call to action, gestures that point to each observer, demanding the full acceptance of the civil rights of Asian Americans as well as the power of artistry over politics.

# FURTHER READING

Armor, John and Wright, Peter. *Manzanar* with photos by Ansel Adams, New York: Times Books, 1988. This book gives insights into life at the Japanese American Internment Camp, *Manzanar*. Through documented stories and photographs of the camp and its inhabitants, the injustice faced by Japanese Americans under Executive Order 9066 is revealed. This publication is especially useful in understanding the reality of Michio Itō's circumstance from 1941–1943.

Caldwell, Helen. *Michio Ito: The Dancer and His Dances*. Los Angeles: The University of California Press, 1977. This book traces the beginnings of Itō's career in Europe, its expansion in New York and finally to its climax in California before his repatriation in 1942. Of especial interest are the historic photos of Itō's repertoire and his dance technique.

Foster, Susan Leigh. "Choreographies and Choreographers," in *Worlding Dance: Studies in International Performance*. New York: Palgrave Macmillan, 2009. This book chapter explores the "othering" and "forgetting" of Michio Itō due to the labeling of him as an international artist which came into conflict with U.S. nationalism. This chapter considers the effects of the racialization of Itō's migration story on his career and legacy.

Warren, Larry. *Lester Horton: Modern Dance Pioneer*. New York: Marcel Dekker, Inc., 1977. This is a comprehensive biography of Lester Horton, the protégé of Michio Itō and the mentor of Alvin Ailey. This book allows the reader to understand the historical impact of Itō's legacy on multiple generations of dancer in America.

# TIMELINE

1892 or 1893 – Michio Itō is born in Tokyo, Japan.

1914 – Japan declares war on Germany; Itō moves to England.

1916 – Itō creates his signature solo, *Pizzacati*.

1928–1929 – Itō's company goes on tour.

1929 – Itō stages *The New World Symphony*.

December 7, 1941 – the Japanese attack Pearl Harbor.

December 8, 1941 – the U.S. government arrests Itō.

February 19, 1942 – President Franklin D. Roosevelt signs Executive Order 9066.

April 1942 – Itō is moved between internment camps at Fort Sill in Oklahoma, and then to Camp Livingston in Louisiana.

1943 – Michio Itō repatriates to Japan.

1961 – Michio Itō dies in Tokyo.

# BIBLIOGRAPHY

"Biography: Ito-Foundation." Michio Ito Foundation, 2014. www.michioito.org/about.

Blumberg, Sarah. "Martha Graham and Isamu Noguchi a Brilliant Collaboration." Carnegie Hall, 2021. www.carnegiehall.org/Blog/2011/03/Martha-Graham-and-Isamu-Noguchi-A-Brilliant-Collaboration.

"Booloo." IMDb. Accessed 2021. www.imdb.com/title/tt0029935/.

Caldwell, Helen. *Michio Ito: The Dancer and His Dances*. University of California, 1977.

Cantú, Aaron. "When Santa Fe Had a Japanese Prison Camp." *Santa Fe Reporter*, February 21, 2018. www.sfreporter.com/news/2018/02/21/when-santa-fe-had-a-japanese-prison-camp/.

Causey, Adam Kealoha. "Oklahoma Base Set for Migrant Site Was WWII Internment Camp." *Army Times*, June 13, 2019. www.armytimes.com/news/your-army/2019/06/13/oklahoma-base-set-for-migrant-site-was-wwii-internment-camp/.

Cowell, Mary-Jean, and Satoru Shimazaki. "East and West in the Work of Michio Ito." *Dance Research Journal* 26, no. 2 (1994): 11–23. Accessed August 28, 2021. doi:10.2307/1477913.

"Decennial Population Census 1940." Census.gov, n.d.

Desmond, Jane. "Dancing out the Difference: Cultural Imperialism and Ruth St. Denis's 'Radha' of 1906." *Signs* 17, no. 1 (1991): 28–49. Accessed August 28, 2021. www.jstor.org/stable/3174444.

"Emile Jaques-Dalcroze." Dalcroze Society of America, May 11, 2019. https://dalcrozeusa.org/about-dalcroze/what-is-dalcroze/emile-jaques-dalcroze/.

"EO9066: Introduction." EO9066. Japanese American National Museum: UCLA Film and Television Archive. Accessed August 28, 2021. https://eo9066.library.manoa.hawaii.edu/.

Foulkes, Julia L. *Modern Bodies Dance and American Modernism from Martha Graham to Alvin Ailey*. University of North Carolina, 2002.

"HIRO-ARTIST." HIRO, 2016. www.hiro-artist.com/.

"History." Hellerau. European Center for the Arts, October 19, 2020. www.hellerau.org/en/history/.

Jaques-Dalcroze, Emile. "Rhythm, Music and Education." *Journal of Education* 94, no. 12 (October 1921): 319–319. https://doi.org/10.1177/002205742109401204.

Riefe, Jordan. "Chinese Artist Ai Weiwei on His Memoir, His Persecution and 'Why Autocracy Fears Art'." *Los Angeles Times.* November 1, 2021. www.latimes.com/entertainment-arts/books/story/2021-11-01/chinese-artist-ai-weiwei-on-his-memoir-his-persecution-and-why-autocracy-fears-art.

Kaufman, Sarah. "The Power of Michio Ito." *The Washington Post.* WP Company, January 22, 1996. www.washingtonpost.com/archive/lifestyle/1996/01/22/the-power-of-michio-ito/eabd30da-5179-4e2c-9f97-1bad1458d27e/.

Kaufman, Sarah. "Retracing Lost Steps." *The Washington Post.* WP Company, January 14, 1996. www.washingtonpost.com/archive/lifestyle/style/1996/01/14/retracing-lost-steps/471eba34-d198-4a0e-b732-233dc4e4470b/.

Kihm. "Incense, 1906." Read, Seen, Heard, April 22, 2009. https://kihm2.wordpress.com/2009/04/21/incense-1906-2/.

Kisselgoff, Anna. "Dance View." *The New York Times.* July 2, 1978. www.nytimes.com/1978/07/02/archives/dance-view-pauline-koners-golden-anniversary-dance-view-pauline.html.

Kisselgoff, Anna. "'Sylvia': A POST-ROMANTIC Ballet to Hear." *The New York Times.* March 21, 1982. www.nytimes.com/1982/03/21/arts/dance-view-sylvia-a-post-romantic-ballet-to-hear.html.

"Lester Horton." Alvin Ailey American Dance Theater. Alvin Ailey Dance Foundation, 2021. www.alvinailey.org/lester-horton.

"Lester Horton." The Dance History Project of Southern California, 2021. www.dancehistoryproject.org/index-of-artists/lester-horton/.

*Martha Graham Timeline: – 1949.* Web. www.loc.gov/item/ihas.200154832/.

McCluhan, Marshall. "The Medium is the Message." In *Understanding Media: The Extensions of Man,"* ed. Marshall McLuhan. 1964.

"Michio Ito." Virtual History. Accessed 2021. www.virtual-history.com/movie/person/6156/michio-ito.

Muray, Nickolas. *Michio Ito. National Portrait Gallery.* Smithsonian Institution, n.d. https://npg.si.edu/object/npg_NPG.78.148.

Nguyen, Hanh. "'The Vietnam War': How Jane Fonda Became One of the Most Hated People Associated with the War." IndieWire. September 27, 2017. www.indiewire.com/2017/09/the-vietnam-war-jane-fonda-vietnam-photo-hanoi-jane-pbs-1201880919/.

"Noh Drama." *Asia for Educators.* Columbia University, 2021. http://afe.easia.columbia.edu/special/japan_1000ce_noh.htm.

Perron, Wendy. "Michio Ito (1893 To 1961)." WENDY PERRON, May 30, 2021. https://wendyperron.com/michio-ito-1893-to-1961/.

"'Pinwheel Revel' Odd.; Michio Itow's Dances Combined with Raymond Hitchcock's Fun." *The New York Times.* June 16, 1922. www.nytimes.com/1922/06/16/archives/pinwheel-revel-odd-michio-itows-dances-combined-with-raymond.html.

Prevots, Naiama. *Dancing in the Sun: Hollywood Choreographers, 1915–1937.* UMI Research Press, 1987.

Program notes for *Michio Ito Ballet.* Los Angeles: Greek Theatre, August 25, 1933.

Program notes for *Michio Ito & Company.* Wolfsohn Concert Series. New York: Scottish Rite Auditorium, February 1, 1929.

Riordan, Kevin. "Performance in the Wartime Archive: Michio Ito at the Alien Enemy Hearing Board." *American Studies* 56, no. 1 (2017): 67–89. doi:10.1353/ams.2017.0003.

Rod, Tara. "Altered Belonging: The Transnational Modern Dance of Itō Michio." PhD diss. Northwestern University, 2017.

Sato, Yoko. "'At the Hawk's Well': Yeats's Dramatic Art of Visions." *Journal of Irish Studies* 24 (2009): 27–36. Accessed August 28, 2021. www.jstor.org/stable/27759624.

Stewart, Jessica. "500 Japanese Woodblock Prints from Van Gogh's Collection Are Now Available to Download." My Modern Met, February 2, 2019. https://mymodernmet.com/van-gogh-museum-japanese-woodblock-prints/.

Stracqualursi, Veronica, and Jasmine Wright. "Biden Signs Order Establishing White House Initiative on Asian Americans, Native Hawaiians, and Pacific Islanders." CNN. Cable News Network, May 28, 2021. https://edition.cnn.com/2021/05/28/politics/biden-asian-american-initiative/index.html.

Warren, Larry. *Lester Horton: Modern Dance Pioneer.* University of California, 1977.

Weisberg, Gabriel P. "The early years of Philippe Burty: art critic, amateur and japoniste: 1855–1875." PhD diss. Johns Hopkins University, 1967.

Weiwei, Ai. "1000 Years of Joys and Sorrows: A Memoir." Translated by Allan H. Barr. Crown Publishing Group, 2021.

Wong, Yutian. "Artistic Utopias: Michio Ito and the international." In *Worlding Dance*, ed. Susan Foster, 159. 2009.

# NOTES

1 Marshall McCluhan, "The Medium is the Message," in *Understanding Media: The Extensions of Man,*" ed. Marshall McLuhan (1964).

2 Yutian Wong, "Artistic Utopias: Michio Ito and the international," in *Worlding Dance*, ed. Susan Foster (2009), 159.

3   Aaron Cantú, "When Santa Fe Had a Japanese Prison Camp," *Santa Fe Reporter*, February 21, 2018, www.sfreporter.com/news/2018/02/21/when-santa-fe-had-a-japanese-prison-camp/; "Decennial Population Census 1940." Census.gov, n.d.

4   Wendy Perron, "Michio Ito (1893 To 1961)," WENDY PERRON, May 30, 2021, https://wendyperron.com/michio-ito-1893-to-1961/.

5   Emile Jaques-Dalcroze, "Rhythm, Music and Education," *Journal of Education* 94, no. 12 (October 1921): 319–319, https://doi.org/10.1177/002205742109401204;
    "Emile Jaques-Dalcroze," Dalcroze Society of America, May 11, 2019, https://dalcrozeusa.org/about-dalcroze/what-is-dalcroze/emile-jaques-dalcroze/.

6   "History," Hellerau (European Center for the Arts, October 19, 2020), www.hellerau.org/en/history/.

7   Perron, "Michio Ito (1893 To 1961)."

8   Jessica Stewart, "500 Japanese Woodblock Prints from Van Gogh's Collection Are Now Available to Download," My Modern Met, February 2, 2019, https://mymodernmet.com/van-gogh-museum-japanese-woodblock-prints/; Gabriel P. Weisberg, "The early years of Philippe Burty: art critic, amateur and japoniste: 1855–1875," (Johns Hopkins University, 1967).

9   "Biography: Ito-Foundation," Michio Ito Foundation, 2014, www.michioito.org/about.

10  "Noh Drama," *Asia for Educators* (Columbia University, 2021), http://afe.easia.columbia.edu/special/japan_1000ce_noh.htm.

11  Yoko Sato, "'At the Hawk's Well': Yeats's Dramatic Art of Visions," *Journal of Irish Studies*, 24 (2009): 27–36, Accessed August 28, 2021. www.jstor.org/stable/27759624.

12  Perron, "Michio Ito (1893 To 1961)."

13  Helen Caldwell, *Michio Ito: The Dancer and His Dances* (University of California, 1977), 55.

14  Anna Kisselgoff, "'Sylvia': A POST-ROMANTIC Ballet to Hear," *The New York Times* (The New York Times, March 21, 1982), www.nytimes.com/1982/03/21/arts/dance-view-sylvia-a-post-romantic-ballet-to-hear.html.

15  "'Pinwheel Revel' Odd.; Michio Itow's Dances Combined with Raymond Hitchcock's Fun," *The New York Times* (The New York Times, June 16, 1922), www.nytimes.com/1922/06/16/archives/pinwheel-revel-odd-michio-itows-dances-combined-with-raymond.html; Caldwell, *Michio Ito: The Dancer and His Dances.*

16  "Michio Ito," Virtual History, accessed 2021, https://www.virtual-history.com/movie/person/6156/michio-ito.

17  Perron, "Michio Ito (1893 To 1961)."

18  *Martha Graham Timeline: – 1949*, Web, www.loc.gov/item/ihas.200154832/.

19  Anna Kisselgoff, "Dance View," *The New York Times* (The New York Times, July 2, 1978), www.nytimes.com/1978/07/02/

archives/dance-view-pauline-koners-golden-anniversary-dance-view-pauline.html.

20  Wong, "Artistic Utopias: Michio Ito and the international," 146; Program notes for *Michio Ito & Company*, Wolfsohn Concert Series, New York: Scottish Rite Auditorium, February 1, 1929.

21  Wong, "Artistic Utopias: Michio Ito and the international," 147.

22  Quoted in Caldwell, *Michio Ito: The Dancer and His Dances*, 91.

23  Kristina Berger (Principal Dancer, Assistant Professor of Dance), interview by author, June 9, 2021.

24  Caldwell, *Michio Ito: The Dancer and His Dances*; Nickolas Muray, *National Portrait Gallery* (Smithsonian Institution, n.d.), https://npg.si.edu/object/npg_NPG.78.148; "Booloo," IMDb, accessed 2021, www.imdb.com/title/tt0029935/.

25  Kevin Riordan, "Performance in the Wartime Archive: Michio Ito at the Alien Enemy Hearing Board," *American Studies* 56, no. 1 (2017): 67–89, 232. doi:10.1353/ams.2017.0003.

26  Cantú, "When Santa Fe Had a Japanese Prison Camp."; Riordan, "Performance in the Wartime Archive: Michio Ito at the Alien Enemy Hearing Board."

27  Sarah Blumberg, "Martha Graham and Isamu Noguchi a Brilliant Collaboration," Carnegie Hall, 2021, www.carnegiehall.org/Blog/2011/03/Martha-Graham-and-Isamu-Noguchi-A-Brilliant-Collaboration.

28  "HIRO-ARTIST," HIRO, 2016, www.hiro-artist.com/.

29  Sarah Kaufman, "The Power of Michio Ito," *The Washington Post* (WP Company, January 22, 1996), www.washingtonpost.com/archive/lifestyle/1996/01/22/the-power-of-michio-ito/eabd30da-5179-4e2c-9f97-1bad1458d27e/.

30  Kaufman, "The Power of Michio Ito."

# CHAPTER 7

# Dance as Healing
## Unearthing Therapeutic Modalities

*Giselle Ruzany*

Before we had oral histories and written language, dance communicated the fundamental emotions of the human experience. In ancient times, dance served as an important part of healing rituals, community-building, cultural expression, and celebration. When people dance together, they transparently share their emotions, physical limitations, and strengths. When watching dancers, one can easily notice their technical prowess, temperament, and even the rhythm of how they breathe. These factors indicate not only how one dances but also the person's overall health. This holistic awareness has been in our consciousness for millennia.

At the turn of the 20th century, dance as healing began to be codified into different systems for growth and healing. In this chapter, the history of this development will be briefly reviewed, and three techniques from different time periods will be discussed in depth. In the United States, Mary Starks Whitehouse from the West Coast in the 1950s; Bonnie Bainbridge Cohen from the East Coast in the 1970s; and Ohad Naharin in Tel Aviv in the 1990s, all conducted profound movement research through which they merged the boundaries of dance and healing. In exploring these examples, I will illuminate differences in dance techniques that were affected by the variance of time, culture, and personal histories. Following a chronological order allows us to compare these dances' healing techniques: Whitehouse's formal and symbolic practice, Cohen's improvisational and technical interventions, and Naharin's dance to find joy and pleasure even when working through pain and despair.

DOI: 10.4324/9781003185918-7

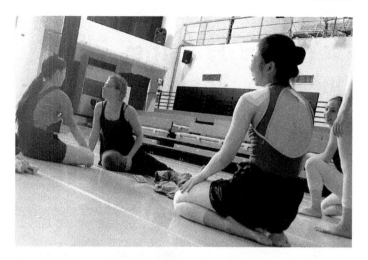

**Figure 7.1:** Giselle Ruzany in conversation with students in Taiwan. Photographer: Jonathan Modell.

Personally, as a Brazilian-American descended from Polish Jews on my father's side and Afro-Indigenous colonialists on my mother's side, dance has been a method through which I integrated different parts of my DNA and thus developed a feeling of belonging in the world. In my journey as a dancer, I was curious about why students sometimes became overwhelmed by their emotions when dancing. A student could become ecstatically happy or sad, and even cry at times. What was this emotional release in their bodies? This question led me from being a professional dancer to becoming a psychotherapist who uses dance for healing. As I practiced as a psychotherapist, I learned that dance could serve as a technique that allows for emotional growth and life skills. As I searched to understand this emotional memory released in connection to dance, I studied Dance/Movement Therapy (DMT), Gestalt Therapy, Somatic psychology/body psychotherapy, and trauma protocols that use the body to heal when verbal psychotherapy was unsuccessful. I will begin with a brief history of how these healing techniques came into being and affected the field of psychology.

# CODIFYING DANCE AS AN EMBODIED PROCESS

The acceptance of the body in psychology has been a slow process. Psychology began to exist as a field of study in 1879, and at that time it was a strictly verbal technique. Nevertheless, the connection between emotions and thoughts that emerged from within the body was already being annotated and codified at a similar time at the turn of the 19th century, mostly by performing artists.[1] The act of moving the body with attention on breath, emotion, sensations, and thoughts is what we call mindful movement.[2] Dance and mindful movement as a process for healing began to be articulated in the late 1800s by performing artists (such as Èmile Jacques-Dalcroze, 1865–1950, and François Delsarte, 1811–1871). Delsarte, who was a singer, developed a method of teaching performing artists to be more realistic by exploring the relationship between inner states and movement. This exploration of mindful movement would influence the opening of many dance centers in the United States and in Europe. In the early 1900s, these movement research centers moved to Hamburg and Berlin in Germany and Vienna in Austria. As a reaction to the industrial revolution, dancers explored less rigid movements by creating dances through sensory awareness and mindful movement in connection to nature and genuine expression (including influential dancers such as Elsa Gindler, 1885–1961, and Rudolf Laban, 1879–1958, and their student Mary Wigman, 1886–1973). Dancers researched emotion and bodily sensations in relation to movement and **expressionist** dances.

During the interwar period, the educated commonly traveled to Africa and India to learn new philosophies and techniques on healing.[3] Ancient dance traditions and mindful practices from African and Asian cultures became a physical lifeline to holistic healing and the body in finding a sense of safety and belonging in European society. Eastern techniques such as yoga, martial arts, shamanic dance healing, and dream analysis were absorbed into dance centers. Through this process, modern dance included practices of mindful movement and sensory awareness in their processes of warm-up and choreography. After the First World War, when much trauma, loss, and displacement occurred globally, leaders in the field of psychology (including Carl Jung, 1875–1961, and Wilhelm Reich, 1897–1957) were influenced by their wives and daughters, who were studying holistic dance and gymnastic techniques, as they concurrently investigated dreams, symbolism, and the body as a source of healing.[4]

These processes of movement research and mindful movement techniques, which came into vogue during the interwar period, influenced fields of study including Somatics (1930s–1940s), Gestalt Therapy (1940s–1950s), Dance/Movement Therapy (DMT, 1950s–1960s), and Body psychotherapy/Somatic psychology (1970s–1980s). In the 1990s, this anatomical sensory exploration returned to the dance stage and dance studio through Gaga. In this chapter, I will briefly define the field of Somatics and Gestalt Therapy and will discuss techniques that have been internationally accepted by the fields of DMT (the Authentic Movement in the 1950s and 1960s), Somatic psychology/ Body psychotherapy (body-mind centering in the 1970s and 1980s), and dance (Gaga in the 1990s to the present).

## ORIGINS OF SOMATIC PRACTICE

The field of Somatics originated in the period prior to World War II and continued to develop after the war by refugees in England, France, the United States, and Israel (important Somatic leaders include F. Matthias Alexander, 1869–1955, and Moshe Feldenkrais, 1904–1984). Without concern for the performing aspect of the arts, Somatics as a field of study was interested in extracting the healing aspects of movement research. The techniques developed in Somatics have the goal of creating an integrated, graceful, strong, and flexible body. Its goal is to free the person's body from any constrictions created by one's personal life story. Somatics fundamentally acknowledges that trauma, depression, anxiety, and hurt are felt and perceived by the body as well as "stored" within it. For example, when a child is abused or rejected, displaced or neglected, a nonverbal memory is connected with both emotional and physical sensations. The trauma remains not only in the mind but also within one's body, until it is understood and then released or transformed in some way.[5] Somatic therapies seek to address the physically imprinted memories that result from trauma.

# GESTALT THERAPY

Dance and Somatics began to influence the field of psychology in the United States and Europe in the 1940s. As World War II raged on, dancers started to collaborate with psychiatrists in hospitals and mental wards. In 1940, Laura Perls (1905–1990), a dancer who survived World War II, became an important figure in bringing the body into the field of psychology as a cofounder and cocreator of Gestalt Therapy in New York City. The formation and evolving field, theory, and practice of Gestalt Therapy will not be addressed in this chapter. Nevertheless, an important concept in Gestalt is embodied relational contact. This concept refers to the philosophical foundation that a person cocreates a relationship with another, through **co-regulating** the relational and emotional experience within each person's body and the environment. In other words, the body in relationship is attentive to the self, the other, and the relational field (the contextual environment). By experimenting with movement in relationship to others and their environment, Gestalt became a philosophical foundation for both postmodern dance and the use of dance as healing.

In my work with "dancing one's ancestral legacy," I use a Gestalt approach by asking people to move from the sensations they find in their bodies when they think of an ancestor, and then to move as if they were their ancestor, and then to move from the relational space that is between them and their ancestor. In this way, a person is moving from an embodiment of the self, the other, and the field, thus creating a choreography of the many aspects of a relationship as it is stored in the body. I then ask the mover to give voice to these movements by creating a storytelling narrative and facilitating the cognitive understanding of the experience of the dance. This process helps people understand the relationship by exploring in the "here and now" of what is alive in their body in regard to their ancestral legacy. This choreographic process follows the process of Gestalt Therapy, where the self, the other, and the field impact the whole organism, including one's experience and perceptions of life.[6]

Gestalt Therapy influenced dancers as well as the development of dancers as healers, including Anna Halprin (born in 1920) and Gabrielle Roth (1941–2012). Parallel to the establishment of Gestalt Therapy, many new psychological and philosophical foundations emerged during this time (including humanism, existentialism, transpersonal psychology, and others). Similarly, between the 1940s and 1960s, dancers began teaching in hospitals, schools for the Deaf, differently-abled children, orphanages, and other institutions of the time.[7] Like Perls, some dancers studied psychology and developed their own theories of how dance could heal mental health conditions. Mary Starks Whitehouse (1911–1979) is an important dancer who began to develop her work a decade after Perls; Whitehouse is one of the first leaders in the field of Dance/Movement Therapy. I will discuss her contributions next.

## PIONEER OF DANCE/MOVEMENT THERAPY

The 1950s was a backdrop for transformation, with World War II (1939–1945) still fresh in everyone's minds and with the onset of the Vietnam War, which began in 1955, psychology began bringing the body back into the process of emotional healing. In the dance world, Whitehouse challenged dance as a performing art by instead using it as a process to increase self-knowledge and self-awareness. She was one of the first leaders in the field of dance as healing who developed a specific structure for movement research; her work was embraced internationally and remains relevant and revered today. In this structure, there are three parts: the mover (who keeps their eyes closed), the witness, and the space. The clear structure and immediate results make it accessible.

Whitehouse was a trained modern dancer and professor of dance at the University of California, Los Angeles. She was also a student at the C.G. Jung Institute in Zurich and a participating member of analytical psychology studies. Whitehouse believed that the body could be a source of symbolic imagery, much like a "waking dream." For example, as dancers move, they might imagine they have wings or turtle shells and, for a time, daydream about being in a forest or dancing with angels. Whitehouse developed her major theory in the 1950s; her disciple, Janet Adler, later called this process "Authentic Movement." The development of her work took a deeper dive after her husband went overseas; she divorced him and was left with two children to raise. She mostly worked with middle-class adults who wanted to get in touch with their bodies. Whitehouse was not interested in dance as performance; rather she focused on the process of moving with what she called "authenticity." For her, authenticity meant improvised movement to be experienced in the moment. When asked if Authentic Movement was a type of psychotherapy, Whitehouse responded that it was a process of increasing self-knowledge and therefore had the same goal.[8]

The Authentic Movement process involves a minimum of two people or two groups: witness(es) and mover(s). The witness watches, and the mover closes their eyes and moves by following the internal impulses and sensations within their body. This often goes on in silence for approximately 45 minutes. It is like meditation, except that, instead of sitting and witnessing thoughts and sensations without judgment, participants do so while moving. The mover creates a dance by "listening" to internal cues and improvising movement that feels authentic to them, without the desire to perform or to be admired. The movements created by the mover are not planned, rehearsed, or drawn from repertoire. The outside witness holds a non-judging role. When participating in an Authentic Movement session, one senses what is happening not only within the body, but also, if practicing within a group situation, in the group as a whole collective. This free association leads to self-discovery. After extended periods of moving, individuals may experience sadness, tranquility, or sensory imagery.

After a session, there is an exchange between the mover and witness. First, the mover is invited to ground and center by journaling or drawing one's experience. Then, the mover verbally expresses their experience to the witness. The core concept is that a witness is not there to interpret but to be a benevolent and non-judging part of the environment. The witness assists the mover in creating a sense of being seen and helps the mover develop an inner sense of unconditional acceptance and belonging. Authentic Movement reflects the culture of the time; the closed eyes resemble the psychiatrist behind the couch; and the free association of movement is similar to the "patient" speaking in a free-flow format about whatever comes to mind. Using the body as the medium for communication propels an important shift in the participant's consciousness and, therefore aids healing and self-acceptance.

Today, this is taught as a Dance/Movement Therapy (DMT) technique, but it existed prior to the codification of DMT. Whitehouse was one of the founders of the DMT association and an important leader in the field of dance as healing. Before I get into the history of DMT, let me share my own experience with Authentic Movement. I learned about Authentic Movement while earning my master's degree in DMT. This technique was part of our first-year curriculum. After I graduated, I did many hours of supervised Authentic Movement meetings. Supervision is a requirement for counselors and has been part of how therapists are trained since the 1900s, when psychology began to train medical students to become psychoanalysts. I would meet with a group of recent graduates, and we would divide our group into witnesses and movers, journal after each session, and debrief with one another. No corrections or advice was given; we just naturally grew in self-understanding and self-acceptance. Authentic Movement is definitely not for the faint of heart, as it can bring up dark imagery and complicated emotions as well as spiritual experiences. The intricacies that arise within oneself and one's imagination can take a lifetime to understand. As a technique of DMT, it serves as an important foundation in forming and educating dance/movement therapists. Furthermore, it is a simple structure that can be easily recreated by a group of willing movers interested in investigating their "shadows," or, in other words, the aspects of their selves they are not consciously aware of. Authentic Movement is recognized as a quintessential DMT technique.

# DANCE/MOVEMENT THERAPY ASSOCIATION

In the 1960s, the United States became the new center of the synergy of dance, psychology, and Somatic practices. In 1966, enough dancers were using dance as a type of psychotherapy and healing practice that the DMT association was founded in the U. S. The culture of the times emphasized community and intensified sharing of research and information. The first members of DMT were dancer-teachers who had been using dance as a healing technique since the 1940s on both the East and West Coasts of the United States. Amid the 1960's inclusive mantra of love and peace, new movement techniques based on moving with less formal dance training and body effort emerged. The idea that dance could be healing and accessible to all was present in popular music festivals from the Monterey International Pop Festival in California to the famous Woodstock Music and Art Fair in New York State in 1969.

In the 1970s, DMT began to provide curricular training in colleges in the United States and in England, and Australasia (Australia, New Zealand, and Papua New Guinea) in the 1980s. Today, DMT training takes place at universities all over the world, including Canada, Israel, and Japan. Dance as healing continued to expand to residential homes for the elderly, after school programs for at-risk youth, psychotherapy private practices, occupational therapy centers, and others. Nevertheless, these organizations now often require qualifications as determined by the DMT association, as using dance with these populations can be challenging. In the 1970s, another wave of dancers began integrating their work within the field of health care. An important and well-known second-generation DMT practitioner is Bonnie Bainbridge Cohen, whom I will discuss next.

## A second generation dancer and facilitator of healing

Cohen (born in 1943) entered the practice of dance as healing from a less structured framework. Her work has been used for psychotherapy, massage, dance education, occupational therapy, and more. In the 1970s, Cohen, a trained dancer and an occupational therapist, developed her Body-Mind Centering (BMC) school.[9] She grew up in New York City, where she had a difficult childhood: she survived polio, poverty, and many life disruptions, including being told to hide her Jewish lineage and living for a time in a foster home. In BMC, Cohen integrated her studies in occupational therapy, dance, martial arts, yoga, movement awareness, anatomy, developmental neurology, relational attunement, and touch into one body of research. Furthermore, she worked to understand movement quality and psychological and emotional affinity as existing within the many layers of human anatomy. Her vast curiosity and interest in healing were wide ranging throughout her life. Among the many possibilities and information one can get from BMC, two in particular are worth mentioning. Next, I will discuss these two aspects: how developmental movement affects neurological development and how one's anatomy is embodied from the cell to the whole organism.[10]

## BODY-MIND CENTERING

Cohen had a gift for explaining and assisting developmental movement problems in babies. She observed a spiral of the spine when a baby was born from a natural birth. The baby would begin life, sometimes startled by cold air, by making a movement that radiated out from the center of the torso, like a starfish, and spread out to the fingers and toes: in a "naval radiation." The baby would also reach with the nose towards the mom's smell and reach with the palate of the mouth to have one's first latch and nursing experience and then push away when finished, finally yielding into a satisfying rest.[11] All these meticulous movements of the cranial-sacral balance were observed, studied, understood, and supported from a nonverbal visceral level.

BMC compares the development of movements of arms and legs to animal evolution, or phylogenesis. In a session, the practitioner helps the participant find the right initiation of a developmental movement (reach, grasp, pull, push, and yield). Developmental movement is an important step in a child's overall evolution, beginning with the head-to-tail connection followed by a homologous movement, in other words like an amphibious animal (like a frog), with upper body and lower-body coordination. The lateral movement (like a lizard) as a homolateral movement, is followed by crawling (like quadrupeds) as a contralateral coordination, followed by a squat (like a primate), with the push of the heels, until the pelvic floor can rise into erect posture. Each movement is a neurological step on a ladder of healthy development. When a child skips one of these basic developmental movements, neurological problems and even the slowing of verbal and reading skills development can arise.[12]

Another area of Cohen's work is the study of "embodied anatomy." Cohen fostered the idea of moving with attention to the bones, muscles, fascia, blood, hormonal glands, and organs. For Cohen, moving through one's bones meant a looseness in their joints in contrast to someone who moves in a muscularly and bound-motivated way. Cohen was an expert not only in facilitating movement but also in the use of touch to assist people in becoming aware of the many layers of their body. By facilitating movement and assisting with touch and imagery, Cohen guided her clients to a deeper awareness of multiple aspects of their bodies in both posture and motion. With more knowledge and awareness, her clients were able to stop harmful movement patterns that had caused chronic injury. Logically, if people learn how specific movements cause pain, they can heal themselves by not repeating them and by considering more efficient movement patterns.

I was introduced to BMC at my undergraduate college. During that time, I spent a week in a workshop with Cohen in Amherst, Massachusetts, and then continued to study it as part of my masters in DMT training. During my undergraduate education, I spent hours in the studio doing my own movement research, imagining my bones and my muscles and pondering such questions as, "What does it mean to move from my lymph fluids versus from my arterial blood?" and "What is the natural movement pulse of my kidneys?" During my master's studies in DMT, I continued studying BMC for its applications to psychotherapy work. Students gave sessions to one another, learning to spot which actions were missing or which fluid or layer of the body could not integrate into their movements. During my studies, I used BMC in my internships working with at-risk youth, the elderly, children with different abilities, preschoolers, dance classes, and even in private counseling sessions. By learning to read different developmental actions and anatomical preferences, I now can see what is missing or overused and help my clients explore missing developmental movements or embodied qualities. This work gives the client more choices in how to embody a more integrated and centered life. It allows me as a dance teacher to pick and choose what to integrate into the class without necessarily following a prescribed movement sequence; rather, it allows for an openness as to what students need in the moment. BMC is complex, but it serves as a philosophical foundation for embodied research.

Outside of the therapy world and DMT studies, new techniques that investigate the body from a somatic curiosity emerged. In the 1980s, everyone in the dance community knew about BMC; a similar form of movement research surfaced in the 1990's called Gaga. This technique, though not officially recognized as a therapy, is gaining popularity because it can be practiced by people of all abilities, from children with different abilities to professional ballet dancers. While DMT and body psychotherapy focus on the research aspects of these earlier techniques' effectiveness, Gaga is a refreshing return to dance.

## Dance returns to mindful movement and healing

Gaga was developed not by an occupational therapist or a psychotherapist but by a dancer/choreographer. In 1990,

Israeli dance artist Ohad Naharin (born in 1952) accepted a position as the artistic director of the Batsheva Dance Company and moved back to Israel. After working as a dancer internationally, Naharin returned to Israel in the midst of the Gulf War, with his wife Mari Kajiwara (a former dancer with Alvin Ailey American Dance Theater). In the film documentary *Mr. Gaga*, Kajiwara is shown having a difficult time adapting to the new culture of Israel, and even kept her clock on a New York City time zone. I can imagine the challenges Naharin faced in choreographing new dances while bombs were falling; experiencing physical pain caused by a chronic back injury he incurred in his 20s, and witnessing his wife's difficult adjustment to Israel. This is the context in which Naharin created Gaga. It was born out of the necessity to heal himself and help his fellow dancers recover from bodily injuries and loss.[13] In that process, Naharin developed his own dance language to describe embodied movement. Gaga resembles a combination of modern dance, martial arts, Somatics, and imagery-based improvisation designed to address the physical, emotional, and creative parts of a person.

Naharin was born and raised among a group of families that lived in a kibbutz community. In the past, kibbutz residents shared the labor necessary to keep the community going, such as farming or working in a factory. The income was shared equally by the community, and the children were raised together as parents took turns watching the children. Everything related to the community was shared. Naharin's mother was a Somatics teacher, choreographer, and a dancer, and his father was an actor and a psychologist. Naharin's childhood was steeped in community living, movement awareness, and functional anatomy, combined with concepts of psychology. Growing up as a natural mover, Naharin became an entertaining dancer in the Israeli army in 1973. After military service, he left Israel and danced professionally with choreographic icons Martha Graham in New York City and Maurice Béjart in Brussels.[14]

When Naharin returned to Israel in 1990 as the artistic director of Batsheva Dance Company, he began experimenting with how to create his own dance language to enliven his chore-ography and assist his dancers in interpreting the work. He used movement visualizations to support embodied move-ment and described dance as living in a "waking dream." For example, during class, the teacher would prompt the movers to imagine that they were in a very cold shower and ask them to explore how an embodied movement exploration felt different from superficially just shaking the body ver-sus living the embodying experience and sensations of being wet and cold. Like Authentic Movement, the experience of the dream is executed from the body, often allowing the dancer to achieve movements that seemed impossible from a technical, premeditated movement exercise. In opposition to the nonperformance attitude of Whitehouse and Cohen, Naharin curated movement to be interesting to watch by using this embodied visualization. He looked for movements that he believed were powerful because he wanted the danc-ers to appear and feel awake and available while performing specific movement qualities. Slowly his dance company began to rely more and more on Gaga classes, and eventually it stopped ballet classes altogether. Instead, Batsheva Dance Company incorporated ballet technique into its Gaga classes. Being an embodied dancer, recreating a movement as if it is done for the first time, is one of the reasons why watch-ing Batsheva dancers is so exciting. Naharin's choreography must be executed with the same intentions of an improvisa-tion's commitment to self-discovery.

Even though there are now Gaga classes all over the world, the original home of Gaga is still in Tel Aviv, at the Suzanne Dellal Centre for Dance and Theatre. It is an enormous room, with huge windows overlooking the Mediterranean Sea. There are no exposed mirrors, and the dancers arrange themselves in circles, forming rings around the teacher for class instruction. During class, students never stop moving; rather, they dance on a continuum, with a soft gaze. The dancers dance as if experiencing a stream of consciousness. Dancers might change the amount of movement or the size of movement, but they always remain in movement, seeking a path of joy and self-discovery. Gaga emphasizes commu-nity and fosters collaboration rather than competition, with students borrowing ideas from each other during the class, and being affected by one another is fully accepted. Like BMC, Gaga asks the dancer to move from different muscular and skeletal layers in the body. They learn to separate the sensation between one layer of "flesh" from another. Gaga incorporates methods like experiencing movement through sensations on the skin over the flesh and under the clothes. Since Gaga is self-directed, when it comes to what your body movement improvises spontaneously, the class has been expanded to every level and ability. Gaga classes can be taken by trained dancers or by nondancers. In the trained dancer's class, ballet technique is interwoven into the exploration of Gaga. Both groups, dancers and non-dancers alike, say they feel a spontaneous healing.

In 2016, I spent two weeks in Israel dancing at a Gaga intensive workshop. This was a transformative experience for me. Gaga contains important elements of Authentic Movement and BMC. There are no mirrors, which forces one to rely on the internal versus external sensations of the body. Classes emphasize imagery and anatomy embodiment, and a live DJ plays international popular music in response to the dancers. Students continuously improvise movement through the assistance of an instructor who gives verbal cues – descriptors of uniquely inspiring images, for example falling up versus down, jumping down versus up, or floating up versus pushing down. Instructors guide the class through movement prompts to allow students to access their own unique anatomy. All the dancers were given shirts emblazoned with one word in capital letters: AVAILABLE. I did not understand why this was done, but, by the tenth day of dancing, I understood that the real magic of Gaga is the act of becoming "available." My body constrictions and holding patterns were released. My breath began to flow in a deep tranquil way, and I knew I would be incorporating Gaga into my personal healing routine and professional work. Recently, amid the global pandemic, I took a Gaga class over **Zoom** with over 1,000 dancers from around the world. Accessibility to Gaga classes has become a global phenomenon, and many are taking advantage of that. In a time of quarantine, Gaga reminded dancers who were stuck in their homes to respect their limits and at the same time find within the possibility of feeling available within their bodies, of embodying freedom and letting go of fearful constrictions. Gaga classes created for me an endorphin-fueled natural high.

One common thread in the history of dance as healing is that moments of loss and grief change the dance from a simple form of celebration and entertainment to a powerful process for self-discovery and growth. Mary Starks Whitehouse, Bonnie Bainbridge Cohen, and Ohad Naharin were all facing loss and uncertainty when they found in dance a path to recovery and healing. This process of dance, done in community and relational connectivity, creates body memories of validation and healing experiences.[15] Dance as a place of self-discovery, through embodied research, can alter one's perspective and consciousness: loss can be healed, fear can be released, and a path to healing one's emotional and psychological difficulties can begin. When someone asks me, "What are you going to do about my issues with the disrespect I witness toward our natural environment, my grief toward my lost tribes, noninclusive politics, and an ancestral history of trauma and war?" I answer, "I am going to make a dance about it." In this personal ritual, I find I am creating my own way to express my desire for healing not only within myself but also for humanity. Dance in early times was used to heal the physical, emotional, spiritual, energetical, and relational parts of the self, the other, and the environmental field. This is what the fields of Somatics, Gestalt Therapy, DMT, body psychotherapy/Somatic psychology and post-modern/contemporary dance continue to do. Knowing this, I invite you to explore the process of moving with consciousness and to use dance as healing into your livelihood. I ask you, "Would you honor where you are and allow yourself to create a movement for whatever is alive in your body today? Would you allow yourself to dance?"

## FURTHER READING

Clemmens, Michael. *Embodied Relational Gestalt: Theories and Applications.* Taylor & Francis, 2019. The eclectic group of

authors and subjects in this book are a testament to the philosophical foundation of Gestalt Therapy, achieving a multiplicity
of individual understandings within a collective whole. The
reader will have a broad perspective of how Gestalt Therapy can
guide a person into an embodied relational experience.

Cohen, Bonnie Bainbridge. *Sensing, Feeling, and Action: The
Experiential Anatomy of Body-Mind Centering.* First Paperback
Edition. Northampton, MA: Contact Editions, 1994. This
book is a collection of articles and writings written by Bonnie
Bainbridge Cohen on essential themes in Body-Mind Centering
(BMC) education. Although BMC has evolved since these arti-
cles were written, the open gaps are inviting and may inspire
students' own embodied research.

Eddy, Martha. *Mindful Movement: The Evolution of the Somatic Arts
and Conscious Action.* Intellect Books, 2016. Martha Eddy edits
and contributes an essential and comprehensive introduction
of the history and theories of mindful movement practices.
This book also describes the evolution of the field of mindful
movement studies from an educational paradigm into a therapeutic one.

Johnson, Don. *Bone, Breath & Gesture: Practices of Embodiment.* North
Atlantic Books, 1995. Don Johnson compiles original writings of
pioneers in mindful movement dance classes, somatics, dance/
movement therapy, and body psychotherapy. This book collection of essays is a must-have for mindful movers interested in the
original writings and the legacy that came before them.

Pallaro, Patrizia. *Authentic Movement: Essays by Mary Starks
Whitehouse, Janet Adler and Joan Chodorow.* Jessica Kingsley
Publishers, 1999. Patrizia Pallaro compiles in one place eight
chapters of original writings by the founder of Authentic
Movement (Mary Starks Whitehouse) and thirteen chapters
by her main students (Janet Adler and Joan Chodorow), who
have advanced the studies to a well-known Dance/Movement
Therapy practice. These original writings illuminate the context in the development of the practice, its analytical theoretical
foundation, and the discoveries made in the beginning stages of
teaching the nuances of Authentic Movement.

# TIMELINE

1800s – Dance and mindful movement as a process for healing begins
to be articulated by performing artists such as Èmile Jacques-Dalcroze
and François Delsarte.

1940 – Laura Perls cocreates Gestalt Therapy.

1940–1960 – Dancers teach in hospitals, schools for the Deaf, differently abled children, orphanages, and other institutions.

1950s – Mary Starks Whitehouse develops "Authentic Movement."

1966 – DMT association is founded in the United States.

1970s – DMT provides curricular training in colleges in the United States.

1970s – Bonnie Bainbridge Cohen develops the Body-Mind Centering (BMC) school.

1980s – DMT provides curricular training in colleges in England and Australasia.

1990 – Israeli dance artist Ohad Naharin becomes the artistic director of the Batsheva Dance Company and develops Gaga.

# REFERENCES

Capello, Patricia P. "Crossing Continents: Global Pathways of Dance/Movement Therapy: The 2016 ADTA International Panel." *American Journal of Dance Therapy* 39, no. 1 (June 2017): 47–60. http://dx.doi.org.ezproxyles.flo.org/10.1007/s10465-017-9246-4.

Cohen, Bonnie Bainbridge. *Sensing, Feeling, and Action: The Experiential Anatomy of Body-Mind Centering.* First Paperback Edition. Northampton, MA: Contact Editions, 1994.

Clemmens, Michael. *Embodied Relational Gestalt: Theories and Applications.* Taylor & Francis, 2019.

*Dance Magazine.* "Ohad Says: The 7 Best Quotes from the Mr. Gaga Film," February 7, 2017. www.dancemagazine.com/ohad-says-7-best-quotes-mr-gaga-film-2307059394.html.

Eddy, Martha. *Mindful Movement: The Evolution of the Somatic Arts and Conscious Action.* Intellect Books, 2016.

———. "The Practical Application of Body-Mind Centering® (BMC) in Dance Pedagogy." *Journal of Dance Education* 6, no. 3 (July 2006): 86–91. https://doi.org/10.1080/15290824.2006.10387320.

Farah, Marisa Helena Silva. "Jung's Active Imagination in Whitehouse's Dance: Notions of Body and Movement." *Psicologia USP* 27, no. 3 (2016): 542.

Feldenkrais, Moshe. *Embodied Wisdom: The Collected Papers of Moshe Feldenkrais*. North Atlantic Books, 2011.

Geuter, Ulfried, Michael C. Heller, and Judyth O. Weaver. "Elsa Gindler and Her Influence on Wilhelm Reich and Body Psychotherapy." *Body, Movement and Dance in Psychotherapy* 5, no. 1 (April 1, 2010): 59–73. https://doi.org/10.1080/17432971003620113.

Johnson, Don. *Bone, Breath & Gesture: Practices of Embodiment*. North Atlantic Books, 1995.

Johnson, Don Hanlon. "The Primacy of Experiential Practices in Body Psychotherapy," (2007):117–125.

Kossak, Mitchell S. "Therapeutic Attunement: A Transpersonal View of Expressive Arts Therapy." *The Arts in Psychotherapy* 36, no. 1 (February 1, 2009): 13–18. https://doi.org/10.1016/j.aip.2008.09.003.

Levine, Peter A. *Trauma and Memory: Brain and Body in a Search for the Living Past: A Practical Guide for Understanding and Working with Traumatic Memory*. North Atlantic Books, 2015.

Levy, Fran. *Dance/Movement Therapy: A Healing Art*. Reston, VA: Amer Alliance for Health Physical, 1992.

Lowe, Richard. "The Early Roots of Sensory Awareness," Fall/winter 2010. Retrieved at https://sensoryawareness.org/wp-content/uploads/2016/04/Fall-Winter-2010PDF.pdf.

Mayer, Christine. "Education Reform Visions and New Forms of Gymnastics and Dance as Elements of a New Body Culture and 'Body Education' (1890–1930)." *History of Education* 47, no. 4 (July 2018): 523–543. https://doi.org/10.1080/0046760X.2017.1410235.

Moraes, Juliana. "Laban no século XXI: Revisões necessárias." *Conceição/Conception* 2, no. 2 (December 27, 2013): 105–118. https://doi.org/10.20396/conce.v2i2.8647705.

Nemetz, Laurice D. "Moving with Meaning: The Historical Progression of Dance/Movement Therapy." In Brooke, Stephanie L. *Creative Arts Therapies Manual: A Guide to the History, Theoretical Approaches, Assessment, and Work with Special Populations of Art, Play, Dance, Music, Drama, and Poetry Therapies*. Charles C Thomas Publishers, 2006. https://search.ebscohost.com/login.aspx?direct=true&AuthType=sso&db=cat05473a&AN=les.2345369&site=eds-live&scope=site&custid=s5702506.

Pallaro, Patrizia. *Authentic Movement: Essays by Mary Starks Whitehouse, Janet Adler and Joan Chodorow*. Jessica Kingsley Publishers, 1999.

Perls, Laura. *Living at the Boundary: Collected Works of Laura Perls*. Gestalt Journal Press Bookstore, 1992.

Vassileva, Biliana. "Dramaturgies of the Gaga Bodies: Kinesthesia of Pleasure/Healing." *Danza e Ricerca, Numero 8 (Dicembre 2016)*, January 30, 2017 (in Portuguese (Brazil)). https://doi.org/10.6092/issn.2036-1599/6605.

Whitehouse, M.S. "The Tao of the body." In D.H. Johnson (Ed.), *Bone, Breath, & Gesture*. Berkeley, CA: North Atlantic Books, 1995.

Young, Courtenay. "The History and Development of Body-Psychotherapy: European Diversity." *Body, Movement & Dance in Psychotherapy* 5, no. 1 (April 2010): 5.

# NOTES

1   Christine Mayer, "Education Reform Visions and New Forms of Gymnastics and Dance as Elements of a New Body Culture and 'Body Education' (1890–1930)," *History of Education* 47, no. 4 (July 2018): 523–543, https://doi.org/10.1080/0046760X.2017.1410235.

2   Richard Lowe, "The Early Roots of Sensory Awareness," Fall/winter 2010, Retrieved at https://sensoryawareness.org/wp-content/uploads/2016/04/Fall-Winter-2010PDF.pdf.

3   Juliana Moraes, "Laban no século XXI: Revisões necessárias," *Conceição/Conception* 2, no. 2 (December 27, 2013): 105–118 (in Portuguese (Brazil)), https://doi.org/10.20396/conce.v2i2.8647705.

4   Courtenay Young, "The History and Development of Body-Psychotherapy: European Diversity," *Body, Movement & Dance in Psychotherapy* 5, no. 1 (April 2010): 5.

5   Peter A. Levine, *Trauma and Memory: Brain and Body in a Search for the Living Past: A Practical Guide for Understanding and Working with Traumatic Memory* (North Atlantic Books, 2015).

6   Michael Clemmens, *Embodied Relational Gestalt: Theories and Applications* (Taylor & Francis, 2019).

7   Fran Levy, *Dance/Movement Therapy: A Healing Art*. (Reston, VA: Amer Alliance for Health Physical, 1992).

8   Patrizia Pallaro, *Authentic Movement: Essays by Mary Starks Whitehouse, Janet Adler and Joan Chodorow* (Jessica Kingsley Publishers, 1999).

9   Martha Eddy, *Mindful Movement: The Evolution of the Somatic Arts and Conscious Action* (Intellect Books, 2016).

10  Don Hanlon Johnson, "The Primacy of Experiential Practices in Body Psychotherapy," (2007): 117–125.

11  Bonnie Bainbridge Cohen, *Sensing, Feeling, and Action: The Experiential Anatomy of Body-Mind Centering* (Northampton: Contact Editions, 1994).

12  Cohen, *Sensing, Feeling, and Action: The Experiential Anatomy of Body-Mind Centering.*

13  Biliana Vassileva, "Dramaturgies of the Gaga Bodies: Kinesthesia of Pleasure/Healing," *Danza e Ricerca, Numero 8 (Dicembre 2016)*, January 30, 2017, https://doi.org/10.6092/issn.2036-1599/6605.

14  Vassileva, "Dramaturgies of the Gaga Bodies: Kinesthesia of Pleasure/Healing."

15  Mitchell S. Kossak, "Therapeutic Attunement: A Transpersonal View of Expressive Arts Therapy," *The Arts in Psychotherapy* 36, no. 1 (February 1, 2009): 13–18, https://doi.org/10.1016/j.aip.2008.09.003.

# CHAPTER 8

# Dance on Film
## From Busby Berkeley to Bollywood

*Kathryn Boland*

## INTRODUCTION

When one thinks of film, dancing might not be top of the list. Yet some of the most iconic film moments have included dancing: Ginger Rogers and Fred Astaire dancing as if on air together, the heroine of *Flashdance* (1983) dancing until her lycra was wet with sweat, and John Travolta commanding the disco dance-floor in *Saturday Night Fever* (1977). Dance on film provides wider accessibility to the art form, as well as a world of new creative possibilities for dancemakers. The art form is a way to bring to film visceral joy and further meaning through the body itself. Dance artists began creating work on film not long after the technology was widely accessible. As both film and dance developed over the 20th century, the separate art forms remained in conversation and left indelible imprints on each other.

## EARLY DANCE PIONEERS ON FILM

One of the most notable times that dance showed up in early film was Anna Pavlova's balletic dancing, in films such as *The Dumb Girl of Portici* (1916) and *The Dying Swan* (1925). Despite her technically imperfect technique by the standards of ballet today, audiences couldn't get enough of her emotionally rich and dynamic performances; in 1916 one reporter remarked "Pavlova is not a woman, she is an experience."[1]

DOI: 10.4324/9781003185918-8

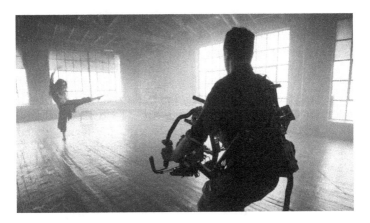

**Figure 8.1:** Photo of dancer and videographer. Location provided by IDEA Lofts and gear provided by Aaron Grasso. Photographer: Brent Barbano.
Source: Unsplash

Pavlova was "the first to open, clarify, and elongate the classical line" – creating that feeling of energetic line through the body that can be so captivating in classical or classically-based concert dance. Her pointe work was innovative, sprightly, and natural to her own body – as were the slight bends in her knees and lack of turnout (which actually came to work to her advantage, as it gave her an appealing "informality and bounce").[2]

Interestingly, given how well known film footage of her dancing is today, Pavlova "was very disappointed in the transfer of her art to film." Of note is that not all of her film work was strictly dancing; "*The Dumb Girl of Portici* presented [Pavlova] in an acting role of melodramatic dimensions typical of the period and threw in a brief solo in tutu at the end."[3]

Nevertheless, prima ballerina-to-be Alicia Markova saw Pavlova dance in that same film at six years old, and later remembered Pavlova's performance to be that of "only a lovely, graceful figure dancing through clouds or sky or smoke." Pavlova similarly inspired and influenced English dancers such as Frederick Ashton and Dame Ninette de Valois.[4] Film dance artists, even at this early stage, were making a long-lasting impact on the field of dance more broadly.

Loie Fuller was a uniquely influential contemporary dance and film pioneer of the late 19th and early 20th century. Footage of her dancing demonstrates the ingenuity and innovation of her work. Fuller released her first film in 1904, and produced three films after that. Other accomplishments of hers include an autobiography and several patents for costuming and lighting technologies (including "underlighting," a film lighting technique used to this day).[5]

Proudly claiming to never have taken a formal dance class, Fuller also challenged audiences to expand their view of "dancing" to one that includes the motion of various aesthetic and energetic components, including lighting, color, costuming, and pedestrian movement. Her performances were something wholly new and captivating; one critic from *The New York Spirit of the Times* described her performance quality as "unique, ethereal, [and] delicious."[6] We see Fuller's creative ethos echoing through dance on film from the mid-20th century onwards, wherein experimentation with various production elements has often created an aesthetic effect that reaches far beyond the dancing body.

Her creative focus of light on moving silk wasn't new when she began doing it, but her contribution was manipulating the light and images that illuminated the fabrics by moving the screen itself, rather than solely by moving the silks, as was already being done. This work, with its own unique complexity, resulted in the continuous creation of varied images and shapes such as butterflies, lilies, spirals, and ripples (some from the natural world and some strictly geometric) – which her film technology experiments uniquely captured on reels. These innovations additionally came at a time when Parisian theaters were converting from gas to electric light, and an energy of innovation around stage lighting permeated the creative atmosphere.[7]

Fuller's work and celebrity persona also surfaced a tension that would resonate through film and through dance art – one between "**highbrow**" and "**lowbrow**" art. Fuller, a former dance hall performer, fully embraced her sensuality, welcomed the masses into "high" art through her universal appeal, and proudly engaged with the ideas and technology of modernity.

Fuller was once asked, in so many words, if she minded performing for working-class audiences – to which she responded that she believed her work could resonate with ordinary people more than it could wealthy art connoisseurs.[8] Here, Fuller's perspective aligns with film as an artistic medium and the way it currently functions in broader society; it brings theatrical art to people who might otherwise never, or rarely, experience live performance in a theater.

Film footage of modern dance pioneers such as Ruth St. Denis, Isadora Duncan, Pearl Primus, and Catherine Dunham also survives, some of which is available on YouTube. Yet in the ways Loie Fuller was ahead of her time, both technologically and artistically, none of these dance pioneers were arguably as significant in the development of dance on film as she.

## BOLLYWOOD DANCES (AND SINGS) ON THROUGH

Film came to India soon after it emerged in Europe, and it was first presented at Watson's Hotel in Bombay. In the audience (amongst mostly British and other European patrons) was Harischandra Sakharam Bhatavdekar. He was so impressed with the technology that he had all of the necessary parts (film, projector, and a camera) imported from England and began showing films across the country, including both foreign and his own films.

Perhaps foreshadowing how Bollywood would evolve to have dance as a central element, many of his films had movement as a subject: boxing, wrestling, circus acts, and animal training. His films included those that appealed to Indian nationals, poking fun at British imperial power, and others that honored the ruling nation. Audiences responded with enthusiasm and delight, and film became massively popular in India; there were cinema halls in every major Indian city by 1910, and it quickly became a staple of urban Indian life.

Yet films shown in India were all American and European in origin (commonly with a cinema staff member translating dialog live), with nothing culturally or nationally Indian in them or about them. Dadasaheb Phalke sensed the cultural demand for film that was distinctly Indian at hand, and – after much fundraising and consulting with other filmmakers – created a film retelling Raja Harischandra's story, from the Indian epic tale *Mahabharata*.

The film was the first of many *mythologicals*, film versions of stories from Indian epics. Phalke and his family (who assisted with creative aspects such as sets and costumes) produced over 100 films. As such, Phalke is today often called the "father of Indian cinema." These mythological films made quite a cultural impact, in large part because Indians could see moving portrayals of their gods, goddesses, and human heroes in the flesh for the first time – not only in the written word or in static artwork. These films still exist with an audience of their own today, such as *Raavan* (2010) and *Raajneeti* (2010).

In the atmosphere of this enthusiastic public reception, enormous production companies emerged – rivaling those of Hollywood's Golden Age.[9] Yet the First World War greatly slowed down production in the Indian and British film industries, while the American industry thrived. American film heads found the Indian market to be profitable, even if they sent old and damaged film reels (having already made the rounds in other markets). Indian producers got these films at greatly reduced prices, for far cheaper than the cost of producing films in the country. Soon enough, 85 percent of films shown in India were from Hollywood.

That trend faded with the "talkies" era. *Alam Ara* ("The Beauty of the World"), released in 1931 and directed by

Khan Bahadur Ardeschir Irani, was the first Indian film with full sound. Following Irani's film, "talkies" were immensely successful, and far more Indian films began to be shown across the nation's cinemas. Films in a native language gave them an edge over the international competition. Indian sound films were making their international mark as well; *Sant Tukaram* (1936), directed by Vishnupant Govind Damle and Sheikh Fattelal, received honors at 1937's Venice Film Festival.

Another cultural dynamic at play was that Indians didn't have many other entertainment forms available, so the market was ripe with demand. Additionally, the weaving together of dance, drama, music, and poetry in these films deeply resonated with Indian cultural traditions, both classical such as *Bharatanatym* and *Kathak* and folk such as *Bhangra*.

These films included increasingly more dance and music with time, according to demand; *Alam Ara* had 12 or so songs, but later films had as many as 40. These films also rarely had a tragic side (with exceptions such as ill-fated love affairs across castes), reflecting much of the nation's philosophical and spiritual stance that life is a transitory illusion ("*maya*"); if that's the case, why not dance, sing, and rejoice? Yet Indian films such as *Sujata* (1959), which told the story of an Untouchable girl raised in a Brahmin family, dealt with cultural issues such as caste with nuance and sensitivity. *Ashani Sanket* (1973) put India on the world map as a cinema powerhouse.[10]

## HOLLYWOOD'S GOLDEN AGE

Early film actors were gradually learning that film acting was a different art form from stage acting, necessitating a different technique. Choreographers were learning the same about dance. For example, one small thing in the camera's view can easily pull a viewer's attention, and film can also pull away much of the sensory impact, weightedness, and dancers' physical absorption in performance that happens on stage. Also. the quintessential film technique of **montage** can dissipate the energetic accumulation that live dance can build.[11]

Film director Busby Berkeley wanted to tackle these problems head-on. He got his start on Broadway, with numerous stage musical credits including the Rodgers and Hart musicals *A Connecticut Yankee* and *Present Arms*.[12] A lavish salary then led him to Hollywood, where he revolutionized the concept of editing while filming. He added influential new approaches and technologies, such as using one moving camera rather than editing the cumulative footage of four stationary cameras. Berkeley's official title was "Dance Director" rather than "Choreographer;" he was as much a cinematographer as he was a creator of formations and movements. In fact, he saw the camera – and not the performer – as the star.

His stage experience might have been part of his ability to create musical numbers with a large and complex visual picture formed by many dancers – like a stage filled with a whole chorus of performers, with each of their movements impacting the performance as a whole. Berkeley also liked using props, from musical instruments to mundane objects like bananas, that could be manipulated to fade into panned-out shots of formations of dancers creating the same or similar shapes. It was a key tool in his toolbox for creating the grand, abstract, and kaleidoscopic effects for which he's most well-known.[13] Aquatic dancing was also in his repertoire, through which Berkeley created spectacular water effects and stages. Esther Williams was Berkeley's star for many of these scenes. His aesthetic explorations, assisted by filming from every possible angle, became even more surrealistic, innovative, and polished as his career progressed.

Berkeley's *42nd Street* (1933), though another in the overused backstage musical genre, reinvigorated enthusiasm for film musicals in a Depression-weary public. The film saved MGM from bankruptcy, and the company subsequently gave Berkeley even more creative freedom and a bigger budget for *The Gold Diggers of 1933* (1933) for which he stepped into the director's chair for the first time. He continued working as a dance director on other films, until he retired in 1962. Swelling budgets for these films forced film companies to cut back on movie musicals in the 1950's, and Berkeley's swansong work was *Rose Marie* in 1954.[14]

The sometimes unrealistic contexts and plots of Berkeley's films do require some suspension of disbelief, but that could have actually been a big part of their appeal in their day; through the widespread economic desperation of the Great Depression and the sacrifices of the Second World War, coming into an entirely different world through cinematic song, dance, and story could be much-needed diversion and catharsis. Also appealing to audiences at the time was these films' insider view of the theatrical world, both in its aspirational quality and its cutthroat reality.[15] One could call that an analog to America – perhaps part of its appeal to viewers on a deeper, subconscious basis.

Dance critic and scholar Marcia Siegel argues that Berkeley opened doors of creative opportunity for dance on film by demonstrating how much is possible within the form, even if it can't offer the experience of the three-dimensional moving body like live dancing can. Scholars, Siegel and beyond, have noted how much of the innovations of Berkeley's visual candy live on in contemporary media, from dance on film to advertising.[16]

Rivaling Berkeley's influence in dance on film in Hollywood's Golden Age was Fred Astaire. The performer, a household name in his career and to this day, made his film debut opposite Joan Crawford in 1933's *Dancing Lady*. His sister Adele had been his dancing partner in Broadway, **vaudeville**, ballroom, satire, and comedy. She left performing for marriage in 1932, leaving Astaire unsure of where his performing career would go next. *Dancing Lady* convinced him that it would be film. His next film *Flying Down to Rio* (1933) was the first time he performed opposite Ginger Rogers, and it demonstrated their unique chemistry as dancing partners. Following films in which they partnered included *The Gay Divorcee* (1934) and *Roberta* (1935).[17]

Through his graceful movement style and overall presence, Astaire became a symbol for smooth, sophisticated masculinity – particularly for young men who wanted to emulate him. Astaire and Rogers, as the idyllic dancing couple, came to represent grace and beauty in popular culture for years to come. They could remain strikingly elegant and easeful while dancing complicated steps. Filmmakers such as Fellini, and later Barry Levinson and Woody Allen, weaved them – as a cultural allusion – into their works.[18]

With changes in cultural conceptions of gender relations, some dancing scenes in these films – such as Astaire's character wearing down Rogers to give consent to dance in *The Gay Divorcee* (1934) – might come off as problematic to modern viewers. Yet the emotional quality in the dancing was generally truthful and anything but conventional. It was important to Astaire for the dancing to deliver the emotion at hand and never stick out as not belonging to the plot.

He also rejected the Berkeley approach of one moving camera, believing that he *or* the camera had to dance. Astaire believed that keeping focus on the full dancing body, with as few shifts in camera angle as possible, allowed even more focus on the work of a single performer or performers than was possible onstage. In the movement vocabulary itself, Astaire mostly called upon ballroom, tap, and his own improvisation. He worked with Broadway chorus dancer Hermes Pan after meeting him in *Flying Down to Rio* (1933), working out both dancing parts and then adding in Rogers (or another partner) later.

The public adored the Astaire/Rogers dancing couple for more than half a decade, until box office sales waned. They worked independently, Rogers in musical comedy and Astaire in musical comedy, until they danced together one last time in 1949 in *The Barklays of Broadway*. Astaire would go on to dance with many more partners in 22 more musicals. Yet filmgoers remained nostalgic for the Rogers–Astaire affinity. Incorporating effects like dancing up walls and always finding new props to use, Astaire danced until the age of 70. Dance aficionados and the wider public alike were in awe of his dancing prowess.

In a wider view, the success of Berkeley, Rogers, and Astaire reignited Hollywood's confidence in the marketability of film musicals. The little dancing phenomenon

Shirley Temple danced opposite tap star Bill Bojangles, as Hollywood's first interracial dancing pair. Eleanor Powell, known for a time as the best female tap dancer on film, also thrived in this era.

Following *For Me and My Gal* (1942), opposite Judy Garland, Gene Kelly was second only to Astaire as the top male dancing star. His style was more weighted and athletic than Astaire's. While Astaire was debonair and suave, Kelly had a masculine temerity. Their camera work styles also diverged; reminiscent of Berkeley, Kelly was committed to making dances for the camera in ways that they couldn't be made for stage, rather than keeping the pure dancing body as the subject of filmed dancing – like Astaire favored.

For instance, "Alter Ego" in *Cover Girl* (Kelly's 1944 directorial debut), had him dancing opposite himself as a representation of inner conflict. Skilled camerawork and timing in the choreography made this effect possible. Following directorial successes included *Anchors Aweigh* (1945), *The Pirate* (1948), and *Words and Music* (1948). Kelly leveraged these films' profitability to try a risky new approach – filming a musical right in New York City streets. The result was *On The Town* (1949), a tale of three sailors' antics onshore looking for women. It had an authenticity not yet seen in movie musicals, and its box-office success paved the way for Jerome Robbins's *West Side Story* 12 years later.[19]

The success of 1948's *The Red Shoes* convinced MGM that ballet could also appeal to the masses. That led the studio to give Kelly free rein to create an elaborate, visually spectacular dream ballet for *An American in Paris* (1951). The final result was an eclectic "synthesis of old forms and new rhythms," as Kelly described it, from ballet to jitterbug to vaudeville.

Following an Academy Award for Direction in *An American in Paris*, Kelly's influence and acclaim was undeniable – even reaching back to his roots in Broadway, where some directors tried to emulate the visual effects he created in films. Despite the influence of those effects, his most well-known numbers are more Astaire-like in filming style – such as "Singin' in the Rain" and "Good Morning" from *Singin' in the Rain* (1952). Kelly also prioritized the story and drama at hand over allegiance to any technique or school of dance. He knew, as he said, "you can't be a truck driver and walk out in 5th position" – that movement needs to follow characterization.[20]

Kelly worked with the African American duo the Nicholas Brothers in *The Pirate* (1948), dancing with a slapstick humor layer to their melange of tap, acrobatics, and vernacular dance. The siblings danced together from childhood, through vaudeville and Broadway before making it to the silver screen. Under the direction of Nick Castle, they made appearances in several 20th Century Fox films – always as novelty acts rather than as central characters. Nevertheless, masters of both acrobatic feats and complex footwork, they had a natural energy and likeability that audiences cherished.[21]

# FILMS OF THE LATTER 20TH CENTURY

Bob Fosse, a choreographer with a knack for making the most of his physical idiosyncrasies, rose up through the Hollywood ranks in the latter 20th century. His jazz dance idiom relied upon purposeful understatement and refinement of gesture to imply sensuality. This style helped build the seedy "anything goes" atmosphere of German nightclubs in *Cabaret* (1972).

Though this dance vernacular was less of a natural translation for tough New York street youth in *West Side Story* (1961), it also worked there – with Fosse taking creative control over the film like never seen before from a choreographer. He received Academy Awards for his work on both (Choreography for *West Side Story*, Direction for *Cabaret*). Rita Moreno played Anita in Fosse's *West Side Story*, bringing depth and courage to her character at a time when many Latinx characters were one-dimensional and guided by predominant cultural tropes.[22]

The "Golden Age" of Hollywood musicals, of which *West Side Story* and *Cabaret* were a part, wouldn't last forever. When Broadway musicals were brought from the stage to film (not an uncommon occurrence), studios would often hire the choreographers who had choreographed the musicals. This trend worked to great effect, as exemplified by Agnes de Mille's work in *Oklahoma!* (1955) and Michael Kidd's film work (*Guys and Dolls* in 1955 and *The Band Wagon* in 1953, for instance). On the other hand, it also contributed to rising production costs in Hollywood musicals – leading to far fewer of them being made in the 1960s.

At the same time, the rapidly expanding world of television entertainment began to keep audiences at home instead of in movie theaters. Studios came to believe that only big-budget film ventures had enough excitement to draw audiences away from their couches and to movie theaters. Innovation and risk-taking waned as these studios feared veering away from formulas known to be profitable, ones that could make enough to cover those high production budgets. These dynamics led to even more frequent restaging of Broadway successes in the 1960's, including *The Sound of Music* (1965), *My Fair Lady* (1964), *and Can-Can* (1965).

Moving into the 1970's, with all of the social and cultural shifts it brought, *Saturday Night Fever* (1977) illustrates the disco era – in which people from various cultural and socio-economic backgrounds found freedom in their bodies by dancing under spinning mirror balls. John Travolta plays a young, working-class Brooklyn man who steps into his power and full presence on the disco dance floor. Travolta excelled in the film, dancing Lester Wilson's superb choreography of disco dances such as the L.A. Hustle and the Bus Stop. Cinematography and direction enhance that work, and viewers get an intimate look into a self-affirming, joyful dancing experience.

That same year, *The Turning Point* made a pop-cultural splash and attracted throngs of viewers to ballet for the first time. The film's excellent dancing, artful cinematography, and commendable direction coincided with cultural mores having shifted to allow the plot to feel more authentic and honest (a number of Academy Award nominations in various categories also attesting to its overall quality as a film). Its themes of secret love, and blossoming youth in tension with twilighting years, resonated with general audiences.[23] The film's star, Shirley MacLaine, was both a life-long dancer and a uniquely talented actress. In her portrayal of diverse characters and in her off-stage public persona, she often defied patriarchal expectations of "respectable" femininity.[24]

A year later came *Dirty Dancing* (1978), in which sensuality in social dancing acts as an intriguing substitute for the verbal communication of love.[25] In numbers such as *Time of My Life*, passion and pure fun enliven a fusion of ballroom, jazz, and social dancing. *Flashdance* (1983), which came five years later, tells the story of a working-class welder who dares to dream of dancing professionally. Though her style of acrobatic jazz is in tension with the highly codified style of the school she has her eyes on, she succeeds at her dream of being accepted there.

*Footloose* (1984) demonstrates similar values of challenging outdated perspectives through dance. A Chicago teen (Kevin Bacon) moves to a sleepy, traditional Midwestern town to find that the town preacher just banned dancing and rock and roll. Bacon's character decides that dancing and music is exactly what the town needs – and, by force of his charm and a string of events (involving the preacher's daughter), the town dances once again.[26]

# FILMS OF THE 21ST CENTURY

*Billy Elliot* (2000) depicts a young boy in an industrial British town who similarly dreams of dancing, and by force of grit comes to be accepted into the Royal Ballet School. The dancing isn't always what you'd expect of classical ballet – more daring, more modern, more eclectic.[27] Similarly, the underlying conflict in the film – with the backdrop of the 1984 Miners' Strike in England – is based more in class and social struggle than in the more personal challenges of many of the era's dance films. The film also shines a light on shifting social mores around gender and sexuality, and resistance to those changes, through Billy's desire to dance rather than take boxing classes – a decision which Billy's father sees as effeminate – as well as how Billy's best friend explores and questions his own gender expression and sexuality.[28]

That same year came *Center Stage*, which would become a cult classic for dance lovers worldwide. The film depicts how a young dancer at an elite ballet school in New York City (modeled after American Ballet Theater's Jacqueline Kennedy Onassis School) – the imperfect feet and technique that lags behind her cream-of-the-crop dancing peers – ends up in a space where she can simply dance and be herself. Dancing in the film ranges from dancers working on rigorous classical technique, alone in the studio, to grand productions involving a more modernized aesthetic and elements of high-energy jazz dance – exemplifying the interest in eclecticism growing in concert dance's "post-postmodern" age.

These films, from the late 1970s through to the early 2000s, illustrate the power of self-expression, following one's heart, and rejecting outdated notions of the body, sexuality, and conventional hierarchies.[29] Parallel with drastic evolutions in shared social mores through the latter 20th and early 21st centuries, the dancing in these films acts as a symbol of a new generation craving change and prioritizing values apart from those of their parents.

*Save the Last Dance* (2001; directed by Thomas Carter) fits into that theme of finding authentic self-expression and rejection of outdated, heirarchically-driven norms, and also many of *Center Stage*'s same teenage troubles in romance and ambition. Yet it is grounded in more multifaceted characters, richer dialog, and more relatable struggles than many of the movies of this genre from the 2010s.[30]

Sara (Julia Stiles) seemed to have a bright future as a dancer ahead, but a tragic accident killed her mother. She must then move in with her father.[31] Questions of race, privilege, and belonging abound as she meets her new – many of them Black – classmates. She becomes close with a few, and even romantic with one, Derek (Sean Patrick Thomas). The couple connects through dance, her learning hip-hop and him learning of her love for ballet. As the film progresses, the characters face tough questions of loyalty and what they want their futures to be.

Though it has the potential for universal appeal, dance lovers might also appreciate how it breaks down fundamentals of hip-hop dance technique, viewers learning just as Sara does – such as the fluid rocking motion that gives hip-hop dance its fluid bounce even as it gets fast and accented. The good part can be the learning process, it reminds us.

*Black Swan* (2010; directed by Darren Aronofsky) depicts a *corps de ballet* dancer's inner and outer world falling apart as she approaches stardom. Through the experience of Nina Sayers (Natalie Portman), we see both the beautiful glory and the dark side of the ballet world; Aronofsky juxtaposes the grandeur of Lincoln Center and Nina's experiences of cracking toenails, bulimic behaviors, and sexual advances of her artistic director.

Nina's hard work seems to have finally paid off when she clinches the Swan Queen role in *Swan Lake*, including both the White and Black Swan. Yet, as *New York Times* Film Critic Manohla Dargis puts it, "as the pressure builds, things fall apart, or Nina does."[32] Aronofsky brings viewers right into the growing psychological darkness of Nina's experience through it all, and we can be left wondering what's real and what's Nina's experience alone. With Nina literally beginning to grow swan feathers and seeing a threat in her counterpart Odile (Mila Kunis), reflecting the plot of Swan Lake, the lines between art and reality also blur.

Light and dark as opposing forces is a prevailing theme, yet in a true postmodern sensibility, Aronofsky demonstrates that such binaries are too simplistic. After all, the womanizing Artistic Director gives her a role that could launch her to stardom, and are his advances motivated by his desire to draw out something darker from Nina for the Black Swan role rather than by his own sexual desires? And Kunis's character might genuinely want to be a good friend to Nina.[33] It's a ballet film for a post-Iraq War, post-Great Recession time when modern audiences are skeptical and tired of simple, black-and-white answers. At a time when many people are beginning to discourage stigma around mental illness, in favor of education and compassion, the film additionally demonstrates the complexity around mental health issues; within the workings of the mind, there are also no simple answers.

Six years later came *La La Land* (2016). The love story of two Los Angeles artists (Ryan Gosling and Emma Stone), it's a film that seems to yearn for something pure, uncomplicated, and rooted in individual rather than broader systemic challenges. Twists and turns through their creative careers and romance take them through a lot yet, ultimately, they land in a place of stability and some form of what they had imagined for themselves.

Choreography from Mandy Moore references classic film dance – of Fred and Ginger, Fosse, and Robbins – in reimagined, modern ways. At a time of concert dance leaving behind wholesale rejection of traditional techniques and allegiance to the purity of singular dance styles, that could foretell much about the future direction of dance on film and dance more broadly.

# K-POP: A GLOBAL POP AND DANCE PHENOMENON

"K-Pop" is a contemporary example of the inextricable link between music and movement, and what becomes of the art forms joined together in filmed performance. K-Pop grew to be a bona-fide global phenomenon in the 2010s, ballooning the South Korean music industry to a $5 billion force. It's part of the South Korean "Hallyu" or cultural wave – including music, dance, and even skin care routines.

Its roots lie in a democratizing of the country in the 1980s and a resulting relaxing of censorship of content over the public airwaves.

The potential for art blending traditional aesthetics with influences from other nations, such as pop and hip-hop, could then grow. A televised weekend talent show culture emerged in this environment, creating a spotlight for national talent. Unlike with most other popular music genres, we can actually pinpoint K-Pop's origin point to an appearance on one of these talent shows. Seo Tajji and Boys performed "Nan Arayo (I Know)" on a South Korean talent show on April 11, 1992. The judges panned the single and gave them the lowest score that night.

Yet the public had a different take; the song spent seven weeks at the top of South Korean billboards. "I Know" spoke about difficult topics in a bold way (teen angst and pressures to succeed and socially conform in a rigorous education system, for instance), free from network censorship and outdated views of what the public really wanted to see and hear.

Dance lovers can point to the place of hip-hop dance in that groundbreaking event, and hip-hop dance – infused with American music video-style commercial dance aesthetics – is still a central part of K-Pop's international appeal. The production value in K-Pop dancing is always top-notch: memorable choreography, stylish costumes, and every count right on-beat.

The success of "I Know" laid the groundwork for South Korean artists to continue challenging norms and breaking barriers, to innovate ways to speak about challenging, universally-understood topics with nuance and in an entertaining, high production-value container. Yet a studio system controls K-Pop and, one could argue, breeds conformity as well as somewhat superficial material (crushes, breakups, and the like).

These studios find talented South Korean children at a young age and put them through a demanding curriculum of music and dance classes, and when – and *if* – they're ready, they'll make their debut as part of an "idol" group (similar to boy or girl bands in American pop culture). Those with true talent and a unique brand might even debut as a solo act. From there, studios churn out hits from these artists with assembly-line efficiency, and production values are always impressive. Making it onto American billboards is a key sign of performers' talent and brand resonating, and international fame often follows from there.

In the face of hierarchical, ethically questionable norms of that studio system, girl groups (such as the Wondergirls and 2NE1) are slowly but surely breaking out of the "good girl/ sophisticated woman" frame. They're speaking out against sexist constraints in increasingly nuanced ways. Boy groups (such as BTS and EXO), for their part, are finding ways out of the "bad boy/sophisticated man" binary to speak about their experience in ways that are more authentic and reso-nate with forward-thinking modern audiences.

K-Pop is also moving away from the homophobia and rac-ism in its past, such as through Holland, the first openly LGBTQAI+ K-Pop artist, making a mark in 2018 and Black artists gaining greater representation, respectively. Heteronormativity and cultural appropriation in the K-Pop universe continue to present difficult questions, but inno-vative artists are finding their own answers in sophisticated ways. South Korea as a nation is also leveraging its native pop phenomenon to portray itself to the world as modern and creative, such as in centering K-Pop performances in the 2018 Pyeongchang Olympics ceremonies.[34]

## TIKTOK DEMOCRATIZING DANCE ON SOCIAL MEDIA

TikTok, a social media platform, is another pop culture phenomenon that closely links music and dance, particularly among those in "Gen Z" (born 1997–2015). Millions of people are creating and exploring their creativity, in dancing and beyond, through the platform. Its litany of possible video and sound effects make it irresistible for creative exploration, and on the viewer side its algorithm makes binge-watching just about addictive.[35]

The platform democratizes creativity by providing a platform for anyone to share dance, music, or something else creative (from recipes to sketch comedy). Democratization doesn't mean that making TikTok videos is quick or easy; it's time consuming for many creators, and resources have emerged to help TikTok creators make high-quality content less laboriously. Not all content is top-notch, either. It's an app originally envisioned as a digital space for collaborative lip-syncing and karaoke, activities stereotypically known for cringe-worthy performances.

Yet some videos, and those with dancing notwithstanding, are legitimately well-crafted and enjoyable to watch. For example, high-profile professional dancers, such as New York City Ballet Principal Dancers James B. Whiteside and Isabella Boylston, as well as several Broadway ensemble members, actively post dance content on TikTok. Dance forms, not always front and center in popular culture, from tap dance to Irish step dance, also get visibility boosts through viral TikTok videos. Dancers of different disciplines sometimes move together on TikTok, as well, reflecting the contemporary dance world's heterogeneous interests.[36]

Apart from highly-trained dancers, "non"-dancers (those without formal dance training) partake in sharing dance content through the platform with such viral dance challenges as "Say So," "Tap In," and "Attention."[37] Underscoring the connection of pop music and movement, the base of these viral dances is most often a popular "single."

Professional or not, content good or cringe-worthy, in the end TikTok is mainly about just having fun. Enthusiastic TikTok users will tell you that much lower levels of ad content, higher engagement with their content from fellow users, and generally low-key "vibe" make it a more pleasant experience to use than many other social media platforms.

Yet the platform is not without its problems – sexualization, racism, sexism, use of users' data, and privacy issues as concerns young users, for example.

Concerning dance in particular, nagging questions of social equity also remain. Lily Kind, the Associate Director of the Philadelphia studio Urban Movement Arts, believes that much of the viral dancing on TikTok "draws from adolescent-girl culture and Black vernacular dance traditions: hand-clapping games like Miss Mary Mack; earlier pop-music fad dances, to songs like 'Macarena' and Soulja Boy's 'Crank That'; double Dutch; and even vaudeville-era routines."

Apart from Black creatives not getting compensation and reputational acclaim for this creative work, this trend can bleed into "'digital Blackface' – a sort of 'twenty-first century minstrelsy,'" Kind says. TikTok dancing reflects the spirit of Black dance in America, she also believes. "It's engaged and playful with the viewer. It's all about improvisational composition and one-upping each other—you did this; now I'm going to twist it, flip it, and reverse it," she affirms.[38]

## CONCLUSION

With the onset of the COVID-19 pandemic in March of 2020, dance on film has been populating the internet far beyond TikTok and K-Pop videos. With theaters closed for public safety, dancemakers across the world have shifted to rehearsing and presenting works through Instagram, Facebook, Vimeo, Zoom, and YouTube. Many choreographers are learning more about, and subsequently intrigued by, the possibilities that film tools offer them in dancemaking. Rehearsing and performing together remotely, though not without notable limitations, can allow artists from around the world to collaborate.

The exact nature of dance going forward is uncertain, but it's undeniable that film will be a key part of that. There's a rich legacy of dance on film for artists to learn from as they explore and create. Just as dance on film always has, the content and aesthetic qualities of their dancemaking will shift in parallel with the changing social mores of the world around it. Just as creators of dance on film always have, they will learn from, and draw inspiration from each, others as well, or decide to chart their own divergent path. There are many paths for the taking.

## FURTHER READING

Billman, Larry. Film *Choreographers and Dance Directors: An Illustrated Biographical Encyclopedia.* Jefferson, NC: McFarland and Company: 1997. This encyclopedic text features nearly 1,000 film dance choreographers and dance directors as well as the 3,500 films to which they contributed choreography and dance direction. Readers can efficiently learn about the work of these artists individually and also piece together a more comprehensive view of the evolution of this art form from the tail end of the 19th century to the end of the 20th.

Branningham, Erin. *Dancefilm: Choreography and the Moving Image.* London: Oxford University Press: 2011. Branningham's text offers both historical context and artistic analysis of choreographic work on film – highlighting the most influential events as well as painting a picture of the evolution of dance on film more broadly. The text also merges choreographic theory and film theory, the latter being a field of creative study that dancers and dance enthusiasts might not know as much on but could benefit from learning about.

Evans, Mark and Mary Fogarty. *Movies, Moves and Music: The Sonic World of Dance Films.* Sheffield, UK: Equinox Publishing, 2016. This text investigates the intersection of music and movement in the medium of film, from the post-War period to the present – historically, globally, socio-culturally, and creatively. Pop culture phenomena such as Bollywood, as well as stylistic instances of dancers creating sound through their performance (such as in Irish dance, Flamenco, and Krumping), are described.

Genne, Beth. *Dance Me a Song: Astaire, Balanchine, Kelly, and the American Film Musical.* London: Oxford University Press, 2018. Genne's text explores the work of these three iconic dance artists and choreographers, and how it both drew from, and came to shape, American pop culture – reflecting American values of pluralism, multiplicity, and the possibility of a better life for any person. Genne also describes how technological advancements and innovations in the craft of directing in conjunction with these artists' works pushed dance on film forward, to ultimately have that culture-sharing effect.

Mitoma, Judy. *Envisioning Dance on Film and Video*. London: Routledge Publishing, 2003. Through the voices of those working in the field, including choreographers, cinematographers, and critics, this work takes a deep dive into the intersection of dance and film. Readers therein can gain a multidisciplinary, multi-perspective look into dance on film, from those who know it in a deep, experiential way.

Rosenberg, Douglas. *Screendance: Inscribing the Ephemeral Image*. New York: Oxford University Press, 2012. Rosenberg's text, both a history and a critical analysis, takes a rigorous and academic look at film dance. Rosenberg calls upon analytic frames, from the psycho-analytic to the feminist to the literary, to probe deeper into meaningful intersections within dance on film – dancer and audience member, dancer and director, dancer (or other subject) and the camera.

# TIMELINE

1896 – Film is first presented in India at Watson's Hotel in Bombay.

1904 – Loie Fuller released her first film.

1910 – Cinema halls are built in every major Indian city.

1913 – India's first film, *Raja Harischandra*, is released.

1916 – *The Dumb Girl of Portici* featuring Anna Pavlova is released.

1917 – *The Dying Swan* featuring Anna Pavlova is released.

1920s – Busby Berkeley choreographs for numerous Broadway musicals.

1931 – *Alam Ara* ("The Beauty of the World"), the first Indian film with full sound, is released.

1933 – Berkeley becomes the dance director of *The Gold Diggers of 1933*.

1933 – Fred Astaire makes his film debut in *Dancing Lady*.

1944 – Gene Kelly directs "Alter Ego" in *Cover Girl*.

1961 – Jerome Robbins directs *West Side Story*.

1970–2010 – Many dance films, often about self-expression, are made with notable advances in dialog and storytelling.

1972 – Fosse creates *Cabaret*.

1973 – *Ashani Sanket* puts India on the world map as a cinema powerhouse.

April 11, 1992 – Seo Tajji and Boys performed "Nan Arayo (I Know)" on a South Korean talent show, marking the beginning of K-pop.

# BIBLIOGRAPHY

Amitabh, Bachchan. *Bollywood – the films! the songs! the stars!* 25–33, 273. New York, NY: DK Publishing, 2017.

Catsoulis, Jeannette. "HipHop and Ballet Cross Paths in 'Step Up'." (2006). In *The New York Times*. Accessed March 3, 2021. www.nytimes.com/2006/08/11/movies/11step.html.

Cortés, Carlos E. "Chicanas in Film: History of an Image." *Bilingual Review / La Revista Bilingüe* 10, no. 2/3 (1983): 94–108. Accessed January 29, 2021. www.jstor.org/stable/25744062.

Dargis, Manohla. "On Point, On Top, In Pain." In *The New York Times*. (2010). Accessed March 3, 2021. www.nytimes.com/2001/01/12/movies/film-review-a-young-ballerina-discovers-hip-hop-and-yo.html.

Dunne, Michael. "Fred Astaire as Cultural Allusion." *Studies in Popular Culture* 16, no. 2 (1994): 9–19. Accessed March 11, 2021. www.jstor.org/stable/23413727.

Ebert, Roger. "Footloose." (1984). Accessed February 15, 2021. www.rogerebert.com/reviews/footloose-1984.

Ebert, Roger. "Save the Last Dance." (2001). Accessed February 15, 2021. www.rogerebert.com/reviews/save-the-last-dance-2001.

Edelstein, David. "Black Swan: A Largely Empty Sensation." (2010). Accessed March 9, 2021. www.npr.org/2010/12/03/131730846/-black-swan-a-largely-empty-sensation.

Gunning, Tom. "Loïe Fuller and the Art of Motion: Body, Light, Electricity, and the Origins of Cinema." In *Camera Obscura, Camera Lucida: Essays in Honor of Annette Michelson*, edited by Allen Richard and Turvey Malcolm, 75–90. Amsterdam: Amsterdam University Press, 2003. Accessed January 15, 2021. doi:10.2307/j.ctt46n2cn.8.

Haskell, Molly. "Shirley Maclaine." *Film Comment* 31, no. 3 (1995): 20–28. Accessed February 12, 2021. www.jstor.org/stable/43455102.

Jennings, Rebecca. "TikTok, Explained." In *Vox* (2019). Accessed February 24, 2021. https://www.vox.com/culture/2018/12/10/18129126/tiktok-app-musically-meme-cringe.

Leivick, Laura. "Miss Brodie's Swan." *The Threepenny Review*, no. 4 (1981): 25–26. Accessed January 10, 2021. www.jstor.org/stable/4383002.

Marshall, Jean S. "The Memory of Pavlova." *Dance Research Journal* 14, no. 1/2 (1981): 85–86. Accessed March 19, 2021. www.jstor.org/stable/1477967.

McCormick, Malcolm and Nancy Reynolds. "Dance in the Movies (1900–2000)". In *No Fixed Points: Dance in the Twentieth Century*, 708–743. New Haven, CT and London: Yale University Press, 2003.

Mitchell, Elvis. "FILM REVIEW; A Ballerina Discovers Hip-Hop, and Yo!" (2001). In *The New York Times*. Accessed March 3, 2021. www.nytimes.com/2001/01/12/movies/film-review-a-young-ballerina-discovers-hip-hop-and-yo.html.

Monroe, Rachel. "98 Million TikTok Users Can't Be Wrong." In *The Atlantic* (2020). Accessed February 16, 2021. www.theatlantic.com/magazine/archive/2020/12/charli-damelio-tiktok-teens/616929/.

Quinlan, Laurel. "The Early Years Remembered." *Dance Research Journal* 14, no. 1–2 (1981): 86–87. doi:10.1017/S0149767700013140.

Romano, Aja. "How K-Pop became a global phenomenon." In *Vox* (2018). Accessed February 16, 2021. www.vox.com/culture/2018/2/16/16915672/what-is-kpop-history-explained.

Scheps, Leigh. "How Broadway Dancer Cory Lingner Perfected the TikTok Duet." In *Dance Spirit Magazine* (2021). Accessed March 4, 2021. www.dancespirit.com/broadway-cory-lingner-tiktok-duet-2649926056.html.

Siegel, Marcia B. "Busby Berkeley and the Projected Stage." *The Hudson Review* 62, no. 1 (2009): 106–112. Accessed January 22, 2021. www.jstor.org/stable/25650732.

Skinner, Oliver. "Rewatching the Queer Canon, Father's Day Edition: Billy Elliott." In *IndieWire* (2014). Accessed April 6, 2021. www.indiewire.com/2014/06/rewatching-the-queer-canon-fathers-day-edition-billy-elliot-214084/.

Sommer, Sally R. "Loïe Fuller." *The Drama Review: TDR* 19, no. 1 (1975): 53–67. Accessed January 14, 2021. doi:10.2307/1144969.

Strapagiel, Lauren. "The Most Popular Viral TikTok Dances of 2020." In *Buzzfeed News* (2020). Accessed March 6, 2021. www.buzzfeednews.com/article/laurenstrapagiel/most-viral-tiktok-dances-of-2020.

Vineberg, Steve. "Busby Berkeley: Dance Director." *The Threepenny Review*, no. 128 (2012): 23–24. Accessed January 21, 2021. www.jstor.org/stable/41550154.

Westbrook, Caroline. "Billy Elliot Review." In *Empire Online* (2000). Accessed March 2, 2021. www.empireonline.com/movies/reviews/billy-elliot-review/.

# NOTES

1  Jean S. Marshall, "The Memory of Pavlova," *Dance Research Journal* 14, no. 1/2 (1981): 85.

2  Laura Leivick, "Miss Brodie's Swan," *The Threepenny Review*, no. 4 (1981): 25–26.

3  Laurel Quinlan, "The Early Years Remembered," *Dance Research Journal* 14, no. 1–2 (1981): 86–87, doi:10.1017/S0149767700013140.

4  Lieveck, "Miss Brodie's Swan," 26.

5  Sally R. Sommer, "Loie Fuller," *The Drama Review*, 55–58.

6  Sommer, "Loie Fuller," 65.

7  Sommer, "Loie Fuller," 57.

8  Tom Gunning, "Loie Fuller and the Art of Motion: Body, Light, Electricity, and the Origins of Cinema," in *Camera Obscura, Camera Lucida: Essays in Honor of Annette Michelson*, 77–86.

9  Reginald Massey, "The Indian Film Industry," *Journal of the Royal Society of Arts* 122, no. 5214: 370–374.

10  Bachchan Amitabh, *Bollywood – the films! the songs! the stars!* (New York, NY: DK Publishing, 2017), 25–33.

11  McCormick and Reynolds, "No Fixed Points," 708.

12  Steve Vineberg, "Busby Berkeley: Dance Director," 24.

13  Marcia B. Siegel, "Busby Berkeley and the Projected Stage," 108.

14  McCormick and Reynolds, "No Fixed Points," 715–718.

15  Marcia B. Siegel, "Busby Berkeley and the Projected Stage," 110.

16  Marcia B. Siegel, "Busby Berkeley and the Projected Stage," 110.

17  McCormick and Reynolds, "No Fixed Points," 719.

18  Michael Dunne, "Fred Astaire as Cultural Allusion," *Studies in Popular Culture* 16, no. 2. 10, 14–16.

19  McCormick and Reynolds, "No Fixed Points," 719–724, 726–731.

20  Gene Kelly and Ron Haver, *Film Comment* 20, no. 6. 57–59.

21  McCormick and Reynolds, "No Fixed Points," 726–730.

22  Juan E. Carlos, "Chicanas in Film: History of an Image," 101–102.

23  Carlos, "Chicanas in Film: History of an Image," 734–737, 741–742.

24  Molly Haskell, "Shirley Maclaine," *Film Comment*, 23–24.

25  McCormick and Reynolds, "No Fixed Points," 742.

26  Roger Ebert, "Footloose."

27  Caroline Westbrook, "A miner's son dreams of becoming a ballet dancer," *Empire Online*.

28  Oliver Skinner, "Rewatching the Queer Canon, Father's Day Edition: Billy Elliott," *IndieWire*.

29  McCormick and Reynolds, "No Fixed Points," 743.

30  Ebert, "Save the Last Dance."

31 Elvis Mitchell, "FILM REVIEW; A Young Ballerina Discovers Hip-Hop and Yo!," *The New York Times*.

32 Manhola Dargis, "On Point, On Top, In Pain," *The New York Times*.

33 David Edelstein, "'Black Swan': A Largely Empty Sensation," *NPR*.

34 Ajo Romano, "How K-pop became a global phenomenon," *Vox*.

35 Rebecca Jennings, "Tik-Tok, Explained," *Vox*.

36 Leigh Scheps, "How Cory Lingner Perfected the TikTok Duet," *Dance Spirit Magazine*.

37 Lauren Strapagiel, "These Are the Most Viral Dances on TikTok for 2020 So Far," *BuzzFeed News*.

38 Rachel Monroe, "98 Million TikTok Followers Can't Be Wrong," *The Atlantic*.

# CHAPTER 9

# Intersecting Body and Machine

## Tracing the Emergence of Dance Technology

*Maria Francisca Morand*

I cannot begin to develop and describe the historical highlights of dance-technology without asking myself why this term has emerged, surprisingly, so recently. The term "dance technology" started to be used in the 1990s, in the more economically and technologically advanced countries, closely tied to computer developments and its use in specific kinds of choreographies. Then how can we trace and build a history of something that seems to have emerged such a short time ago? What background do we see in the history of dance that could reveal this historical trajectory up to what we call "dance-technology?" In order to begin this journey, I believe we must define, or at least, choose approximations to certain concepts that are implicit in this compound term. Technology is an extremely broad concept; it can refer not only "to a body of tools available to humanity at any given point in time," as defined by Mads Haahr (2004), but also to processes that make possible the intervention and transformation of our environment, implying the cross between scientific knowledge and practical purposes.[1] The development of technology is fully intertwined with human history; it reveals not only the advances and developments of the material capacities of different societies, but also reflects their needs and beliefs. So, a society's culture, behavior, and attitudes are constantly molded by the technologies that they use.

This is no different for the history of art; we cannot conceive of art without technology. The relationship between art, science,

DOI: 10.4324/9781003185918-9

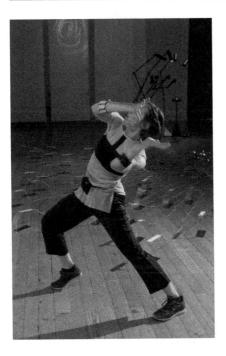

**Figure 9.1:** From *Fragile Intersections* (2019), from Emovere Project. Photographer: Gonzalo Donoso.

and technology has been unfolding since the first artistic expressions, but in the last centuries of our history this relationship has become more intense and intertwined. Today we see hybrid expressions such as art-science and art-technology while it has become common to talk of "interdisciplinary" and "**transdisciplinary**" creation and research. These forms of creation have transformed the idea of what art can be, so that we see in the intersection of these disciplines the emergence of unconventional expressions that challenge perceptions of the world. In this hybrid area of the arts, resides dance-technology where artistic discourse and language are inseparable from the forms of technological production.

The definition of this new field of dance includes a series of trends and ways of connecting, either the body and/or the movement, with other areas – science, digital arts, cinema, engineering, medicine, telecommunications, etc. – that, in the search for new resources and combinations, provide the possibility of transgressing the limits of representations, by altering perception and consciousness. These new forms include dance video, interactive dance with the capture of movement for the stage and internet and CD ROM applications for recording, storage, and dance education, among the most important expressions.

At the heart of what dance-technology implies, this intersection between body and machine is where we find the root itself of what technology is. Today it is hard not to think of ourselves as technological bodies, especially in highly technologically developed civilizations; the distinction between the corporeal and the mechanical is hard to define; technology penetrates us, pierces us, and integrates into our bodies in such a way that it defies the notions of what being human really is. The implications of the "devices," "machines," and "artifacts" that help us to carry out tasks that are difficult or impossible for a "natural" body to perform at the same time change our perception and the way human beings understand and operate in the environment. This is one of the most productive relationships for dance-technology.

> This technological advent changes not just the devices but also promotes a new configuration of body because the interplay between world and human beings is responsible for the embodiment process. It means that different experiences between person and environment inscribe different embodiments, and that different bodies make different dances. This is not meant in a deterministic way but is due to contingencies and unexpected occurrences emerging from the environment. According to this point of view everybody has a 'technological body.'[2]

## DANCE-TECHNOLOGY AND INTERACTIVITY

The emergence of dance-technology as a specific current in the '90s occurred during the development of, and access to, relatively low cost computer devices, together with the sophistication of virtual communications platforms through the internet. The development of technologies such as "Motion Capture" and software such as "LifeForms"[3] enabled the experimentation and integration of digital projections onto the stage, reformulating space and visuality in relation to the dancers on the stage, as well as providing new possibilities for recording and analysis for creation in dance. LifeForms (later DanceForms) developed in the collaboration between Merce Cunningham and Thecla Schiphorst, led Cunningham to expand his movement vocabulary through the software and use it in a number of choreographies between 1990 to 1999.[4,5] In BIPED (1999), one of Cunningham's highlights, he combines motion capture, animation, and DanceForms, by trespassing the movement phrases to animated figures, which were later projected onto a screen that covered the front of the stage, creating a visual dynamic scenario to the live dancers that moved behind.[6]

The interrelation with the media technologies of that time (and which have continued developing at lightning speed during this century) enabled the creation of interactive works, where devices such as software, sensors, digital and infrared cameras, etc., have helped to generate new stage forms where the dancers' bodies become one of the devices that manipulate the visual and sound materials, creating an interactive and/or immersive system.

These new technological possibilities influence not only the way in which dance is seen, but also how it is constructed, develops in space, builds new scenes, and relates to the spectators. "Dance with technological mediation searches for an organic interactivity in a symbiotic way, in which all elements modify and interchange with each other. It's not a mere question of illustration or décor."[7] This statement by Ivani Santana, Brazilian dancer and media artist, summarizes another component of dance-technology: "interactivity." More than just using digital media to compose new visualities and sounds for the stage, the interaction of the bodies of the dancers and spectators develops a language through a corporeal meeting with the technology, a dialog where unpredictability becomes an essential part of the spirit and the aesthetic of the interactive artistic creation.

In the broadest sense, interactivity describes an active relationship between two or more people and/or objects. Mainly used in the theory of the new media and technological communication, interactivity is opposed to a passive relationship between sender and receiver, provided by older media such as television and radio. Specifically, it refers to the ability of a technological medium (generally a computer) to modify its response or control decisions when faced with the emission from one person or a group of people, within the limitations of its language and design. We could say, then, that interactivity is a type of relationship that makes a system's behavior modify the behavior of another, which is reflected in a "tension" between control and freedom: the dilemma of how much will the system try to control the person's activity and/or degree of liberty. Another characteristic of interactivity is that it occurs in real-time, where there is also a feedback loop between the user and the technological medium, which is able to modify future behavior in relation to exchanges of prior information. So, the user and the technological medium become participants, mutually feeding off their respective behaviors. The interactivity is expressed complexly in technological systems with intelligent forms of communication, that is, that are designed to give less predictable responses (**Artificial Intelligence** – AI).

The process of interactivity is based on the body-machine relationship, integrating the dancers in the creation of the work, that is generated by a close and dynamic dialog between a complex system of devices and a multidisciplinary team of collaborators. In this way creation in dance-technology with interaction has very unpredictable elements where the inter- and transdisciplinary collaboration demands a horizontal relationship between the different constituents of the creation; actors, dancers, choreographer, visual and sound artists, engineers, and technicians who are generating the platform where all the ideas and artistic materials meet at the same time as the idea of authorship blends into this collaborative dialog. Even in immersive interactions, the audience also becomes part of this intricate creative process, making artistic decisions, always within the limits provided by the technological design.

Interactive creation requires the design and programming of an unstable system, which makes it more unpredictable, but also provides greater possibilities of creating a diversity of artistic materials. The feedback process between the dancers and the system creates relationships in real-time between the different stage elements, enabling the dancers and/or spectators to modify the visual space and transform sound; movement is captured and reformulated into other forms and materials, reconfiguring the perception of the movement and blurring the lines between the body and its surroundings. As this relationship between the body and technology expands, distorts, and deforms our sound and visual experience, the dancer's body is reconfiguring its corporality while developing the ability to improvise and create with the forms' external space which it could not do naturally. The choreography is then an emergence between body and system; the work is based not only on the dancer's kinetic abilities, but also on their capacity to reorganize their perceptive, cognitive and sensitive, visual and sound, internal and external experience, while becoming part of this new technological organism.

The greater the complexity of the formal elements involved in the interaction, the more difficult is their functional legibility. Nevertheless, the development of formal possibilities is accompanied by the expression of the interaction. This expression occurs first with the conversational interaction between the subject and the digital media. "The idea that expression may be less about exchanging meanings and more about ways of establishing meanings…. In this context (interaction) expression appears as a constructive element of the ability to interact."[8] This interactive expressive process is characterized by the subject's corporeal mechanisms when it finds and uses the "affordance" provided by the situation. Therefore, the flexibility presented by the interactive design may be critical to the emergence of expressive material in the interactive creative processes.

The factor of expression in the interaction had already been noted by David Rokeby in the experiments with VNS

(Very Nervous System), one of the first computer interactive systems between movement and sound. He explained that the subjective and corporeal factor is one of the most important in the creative process, where the quality of the result depends on the possibility of entering into a conversational flow with the system:

> ...they allow themselves to respond spontaneously to the music of the system, it is they who are played by the installation. This approach involves opening oneself to suggestion, allowing the music of the system to speak back through one's body directly, involving a minimum of mental reflection, and thus tightening the feedback loop as much as possible. This sort of situation reinforces the higher frequencies and dampens the lower ones... Among those who approach the installations in this manner I often observe people taking responsibility for perceptual errors that the system's software makes, unconsciously justifying these mistakes by deflecting their intended gesture into harmony with the system's response; conversely, they will often attribute manifestations of their own intelligence to the system.[9]

So, in order to follow the trail of dance technology, we must look at the artists of dance who considered the body-machine relationship to be an important part of their artistic discourse. We will see in these milestones how the artists aimed to propose a new body of dance: a body that produces its dance in this "interactive," interdisciplinary, and transformative dialog with the technology of its time, displaying with their art innovative relations with the environment as well as new paradigms about human evolution.

## WHEN DANCERS USED TO FLY

The flying machines used on stages at the end of the 18th century in France can be considered one of the first "human-machine" used in dance. This technology was later successfully introduced in London and Russia, used to produce a magic effect in specific parts of ballet performance. Although they were not his invention, Charles Louis Didelot (1767–1837), French choreographer, popularized the use of cables, corsets, and movable wings, making the dancers fly at climactic moments in his works. He was possibly inspired by the manipulation of puppets or also by images from engravings depicting cupids and winged beings. This machinery intensified the effect of suspension that he needed to portray in otherworldly characters like cupids, nymphs, or fairies, allowing them to rise up on their toes before being removed from the stage in an impressive illusory flight. Didelot achieved the greatest sophistication of his technology in London, where "the sheer amazement and delight of the British public bears comparison with the world's comments while watching the first moon landing, in the presentation of his ballet L 'Amour Venge."[10]

However, it would be in his ballet *Flore et Zéphire* (1796), considered his most sublime work, where Didelot would produce such an effect in his staging, that it would become the precedent for the light, soft, and delicate figures that characterized romantic ballet. "One of the most captivating entertainments of the kind we have ever witnessed. By an airiness of fancy, he makes all his personages literally fly- for they are borne on the bosom of the air, in a very new and extraordinary manner."[11] While somewhat risky for the dancers, Didelot's technological device built a supernatural and fantastic body that encouraged the spectators to commit themselves to the ballet's argument and its characters. But the most important aspect of the machinery is the impact on the ideal of corporality that the ballet would continue developing over several decades; the ethereal, weightless body, always light and delicate, of the romantic dancer. So, Didelot and his technology are part of the construction of the "dancer," bringing the ideals of lightness and suspension expected in a virtuoso body of the dance to the limit. The device did not last long; it was too dangerous and did not provide greater possibilities of expression for those who were suspended. But without doubt it became the precedent for another dance body technology that has determined ballet's vocabulary: the pointe shoe.

# THE SERPENTINE DANCES OF LOIE FULLER

In 1892 the North American Loie Fuller (1862–1928) burst into Art Nouveau Paris with her "Serpentine dances," an innovative spectacle of lights, movement, and enormous silk costumes.[12] Her technological choreographies are the expression of a mix of disciplines, stage forms, expansion of the dance, and the possibilities of representing the body by a dialog with the new technologies of her time. Her work reveals the complexity of the historical moment, when the industrial era's enormous technological advances transformed society by leaps and bounds. Choreographer, dancer, actress, businesswoman, playwright, set designer, light technician, scientist, and inventor, her staging is the link between theatre, vaudeville, modern dance, and visual performance. Fuller's shows were characterized by the projection of lighting effects from lamps and spotlights on costumes made with huge amounts of silk that were manipulated with the aid of bamboo and aluminum rods, in order to generate highly impressive stage illusions. With an extraordinary ability for invention and a highly artistic sensibility, Fuller experiments with gas and electric lamps, cutting edge technology for the time, creating and patenting the use of chemical salts and gases for stage lighting and for her dancers' costumes.

From the first experiments with her technological gadgets, *La Loie*, as she was known in Paris, discovered that the impact arose from the thousands of movements created by the silk as it was manipulated, together with the visual effect produced by the projection of different colors onto the silk. The choreography lies not in the dancing skills of her body nor in the emotion that moves it; the new dance and its vocabulary emerges from the meeting of this body with the "machinery" of lights and silk, a vocabulary made of sinuous, vibrant, lustrous pleats that blur together in a dark space that illuminates the translucent choreography. Her work reformulates the limits of a conventional dance discipline, and rather than representing a body on stage, she displays a body that appears devoid of its material support. Hence, Fuller places motion on stage through a complex understanding of the technical apparatus and its relation to visual spatiality, where "[e]ach movement of the body was expressed in the folds of silk, in a play of colors in the draperies that could be mathematically and systematically calculated."[13]

In Fuller's choreography, the body in movement and the technology are based on a single mutating image and depending on the exact manipulation of the lighting device and the forms taken by the silk; the body dissolves in its interactive dialog, where split, multiplied, and reconfigured it emerges with a new appearance while the simple and dark space that contains it becomes more complex. A body that is not only a body; a body that in its encounter with technology can seem like water, lilies, butterflies and violets, typhoons and volcanoes, until it turns into an abstract scenery of undulating lights and colors.[14]

## OSKAR SCHLEMMER'S SPATIAL DANCES

Despite the Weimar Republic's (1919–1933) political instability, art and intellectuality experienced one of the most creative and innovative periods of Germany's history. In dance we find the development of modernism, led by Rudolf Laban and the design of the Bauhaus School (1919–1933), that set the foundations of what we know today as industrial and graphic design. Bauhaus established the synthesis between art and technology that empowered the creation and concept of "total art," or *Gesamtkunstwerk*, as an ideal that expressed a new man in a harmonious relationship with his environment, characterized by great scientific, technological, and industrial development in early 20th-century Europe. The positive view of the Bauhaus in the face of technology also reflected Weimar Germany's need to overcome its moral and material collapse following World War I. Although the Bauhaus school's focus was on graphic and objects design, one of the most important workshops was theater one, directed by Oskar Schlemmer, painter, sculptor, and choreographer, where in accordance with the Bauhaus ideas about the fusion of light, sound, color, and movement, he put the body and its relation to space and form in the center of his creation. Schlemmer thought of space as a living entity that could be experienced through sight as well as through touch, while also being abstract and consisting of a complex geometric net. In full agreement with these ideas, Laban, who as well as choreography, had studied architecture, developed one of the 20th century's most important theories of dance. He established that space, as well as being a living entity, is dynamic and is formed along with the body's movement and that the "trace forms" that arise from this relationship follow the mathematical and mechanical laws in which the human being is immersed. Schlemmer and Laban, who saw a direct relation between science and art, held that a human being's "harmony" lay in the relation between his organicity and the surrounding environment. Schlemmer describes the organic body, with its internal functions and movements, as a response to physical laws that can be synthesized in mechanical and mathematical ideas. In his book *Choreutics*, Laban presents a study of progressive sequences that express different ways in which the body, through movement, generates dynamic forms that were inspired by geometry and musical scales. His "Space Harmony" proposes the union of body, space, and movement, an expression of the individual's deliberate dialog and inner world with the surrounding space or environment. So, space also provides possibilities for movement as the subject's intentions change.

Schlemmer, meanwhile, refers to the synthesis between space and body, "Man as Dancer," or *Tänzermensch*, where "He obeys the laws of the body as well as the law of space; he follows his sense of himself as well as his sense of embracing space."[15] The concept of Man as Dancer synthesizes Schlemmer's ideal balance between human being and environment, a harmony that is also created with technology. Laban sees in the body itself and its movement how human beings achieve this harmony. Schlemmer expands on Laban's ideas through technology, recognizing that in the relationship with our objectual world and in the meeting and positive and playful appropriation of technology we can understand our capacities and sense of the human. Schlemmer also described mechanization as "the inexorable process which now lays claim to every sphere of life and art. Everything which can be mechanized is mechanized. The result: our recognition of that which cannot be mechanized."[16]

In his workshop Schlemmer and his students designed voluminous costumes to generate a perception of space on the body of the person using them and on whom the phenomenon was observed. Like corporeal technological devices, these costumes made the performers negotiate their bodily possibilities in relation to the space they were building with the body's movement. We can find a good example in Pole (or Stick) Dance (1927), where the performer appears dressed in black with 12 rods attached to his body. A clear relation between the organic geometry of the human body and the surrounding abstract geometry emerges in the interaction with this interphase technology, created by the performer's extremities extended by the almost two meter long rods.[17] In this work, "where the organic and the mechanical could be rejoined, or, more precisely, where mechanics could be made organic and rendered crystalline," the body can constantly adapt itself to the technology that envelops it.[18] The movement of the technological costume produces a construction of space that would not be possible with the body alone; it opens it to go beyond the human form's limits, making this technological body and the surrounding environment become synthesized simultaneously into a dynamic, geometric, mechanical, and organic image. Body and space are fused into a technological entity. But at the same time, in this technical-spatial encounter, the subject-performer, in his conscious productive process, can perceive his body's limits and possibilities during the interactive technological dialog; the technology as a medium and a reflection of human existence.

## *VARIATIONS V'S* INTERACTIVE SYSTEM

*Variations V* (1965), an experimental multimedia work that combined dance, music, technology, and video projections, is not only an exceptional example of technological artistic interaction, but also an expression of an historic process where technology experiences one of the 20th century's most accelerated moments, mainly in the United States and the Soviet Union.[19] Art undergoes its own revolutions, as an expression and part of the violent social changes in the west (student protests in Europe and the civil rights and Vietnam war movements in the United States, among others), while science and technology, with the arrival of man on the moon, the creation of the internet, the first industrial robot, the first personal computers, the laser beam, and the first heart transplant, transform how we communicate and understand our universe and our body. Scientific theories, like systems theory and cybernetics, directly related to the evolution of artificial intelligence and robotics, penetrate deeply into the arts and culture, to influence the way in which we develop interactive works to this day. Systems theory was first proposed by the biologist Ludwig von Bertalanffy, as a new way to study life or living systems from a holistic perspective. Opposed to reductionism, a system is defined as a group of interacting, interdependent elements that form a complex whole, with a prevalence of dynamic, ever-changing processes of self-organization, growth, and adaptation behaviors. Considered rather a philosophical perspective of life, Systems Theory found in Cybernetics a technical foundation to study the dynamics of relation inside of systems. Cybernetics is a:

> transdisciplinary branch of engineering and computational mathematics. It deals with the behavior of dynamical systems with inputs and how their behavior is modified by feedback. The term was defined by Norbert Wiener in 1948 as 'the scientific study of control and communication in the animal and the machine.'[20]

The articles *SYSTEMS ESTHETICS* (1968) and *Real Time Systems* (1969) by Jack Burnham, gather ideas that were being developed in the arts and that greatly influence how art is generated with technology, by instilling ideas arising from cybernetics and systems theory. Among these ideas are: the relation between the organic and the inorganic, the symbiosis between man and machine, real time processing and the dynamics of interaction, where the "observer" is included in the phenomenon's results. While focusing on the process more than on the product, on behavior more than on the objects themselves, the paradigms of these theories have a big influence on ideas such as the randomness of, and search for, forms of "generative" artistic production. Because of the variety and instability of the factors at play, the work presents organic behaviors when able to evolve in several and new directions. Procedures such as chance and the inclusion of spectators as participants in the works (as part of the system) will become experimental practices that characterize the artistic movements occurring at this time, such as Fluxus and happenings, and that will be expressed by new dance in the United States. In 1966, a group of artists (dancers, musicians, and visual artists) and engineers from Bell Telephone Laboratories in the United States, organized the project "9 evenings: Theatre & Engineering," where a series of experimental installations and stagings were exhibited in New York, in the 69th Regiment Armory, October 13–23, resulting from an interdisciplinary collaboration that "opened new ways to understand the relationship between bodies and machines, adapting technology to bodies' movements and vice versa."[21]

One year earlier, *Variations V* was presented at New York's Philharmonic Hall, with responses that ranged from fascination to disgust, but "none responded with apathy. There may have been some few who did not like it," wrote Patricia Werle in the *Lexington Leader*, "but they will never forget it."[22] The stage setting consisted of two sound systems designed by the composers John Cage and David Tudor which reacted to the movement of the seven dancers from the Merce Cunningham company: Cunningham himself, Carolyn Brown, Barbara Dilley Lloyd, Sandra Neels, Albert Reid, Peter Saul, and Gus Solomons. The staging technology, installed by engineer Billy Klüver, included a protocells system based on 12 Moog antennas, which triggered sounds each time the dancers crossed the beams of the stage lights. The sounds came from the activation of tape-recorders and short-wave radios. Improving the overlay of elements and generating this technological human collage, the staging was interrupted by filming from Stan Van der Beek and distorted television images by the visual artist Nam June Paik, which were projected on large screens at the back of the stage. Although Cage and Cunningham had been exploring for several years the relationship between dance and music, in *Variations V* they generated a system where sound and movement were intimately connected through technology, and the dancers performed as co-composers with the musicians who operated the electronic equipment. At the same time, the work's sound influenced their movement and their actions, as well as the stage space.

> In this regard the work was both successful and groundbreaking. By superimposing the in-puts of an increasingly large number of imaginative personalities, Cage and his colleagues created a work with so many collaborators and such intricate linkages that each participant could influence the sound, but none could control it.[23]

## PRESENT TO FUTURE?

At the turn of the 20th and 21st century, the expansion of interactive technological dance included the creation of specific dance software programs, together with the chance to relate bodily by long distance through the internet, and the use of immersive technologies, such as Virtual Reality (VR) and Expanded Reality (XR) that proposed new compositional strategies for the stage. A growing number of companies and artists began to experiment with devices and interfaces for the stage, but also artistic groups from countries leading technological advances worldwide, were developing their own interactive software with engineers and programmers.

Important examples of software for manipulating the stage media environment are Isadora software, from Troika Ranch and Eycon from the intermedia performance group Palindrome. These interactive environments may involve just the performers or may include the spectators, which means designing interactive ways to integrate in a single event, complex stimuli produced by "expert" subjects together with those who are dealing with this kind of technology for the first time.

In the first, we find, among very impressive examples, the iconic and spectacular *Glow* (2006), a solo interactive dance by Australian choreographer Gideon Obarzanek, (at the time, artistic director of Chunky Move) who in collaboration with the German software designer Frieder Weiss, (also the creator of Eyecon) presented the life cycle of a new being, a cybernetic creature who emerges from the relationship with a machine.[24] But above all, *Glow* is an extraordinary example of an interactive dance work, where body, dance, and technology dialog with the same expressive power, enabling the creation of a work that transcends its technological and dancist materials.

The technology is based on an interactive system of tracking movement with an infrared video camera and Kalypso software, created by Weiss. This system generates visual effects that, reacting to the body's contours, generates images that can morph into and mix with them, creating a flexible structure for the duration of the performance. The interaction allows the relation between the dancer and the lighting environment to generate dynamic, flexible relationships that make each performance maintain the tension and the intention of what is alive and interdependent. "The relationship of the digital pixel environment to the performer varies from being an illustrative extended motion of their movement, a visual expression of internal states, and also a self-contained animated habitat."[25]

The impressive light interaction with the support of the musical composition by the Australian Luke Smiles (with additional music by Ben Frost), generates the metaphor of a techno-hybrid body, a new form of life that expresses its tensions and internal mutations in a constantly changing environment. *Glow* submerges in an existentialist solo performance about human evolution, where this new entity, at times sensual and at other times grotesque, appears to be a body that does not want to be defined; taking on animal-like forms, at times plant-like and, occasionally, supernatural, revealing the drama of this new human's internal tensions during its transformation. The futuristic lighting dialog travels through several atmospheres, where the light follows the dancer's movements, fuses with them, to finally appear as another entity with its own life.

> The seamless joint venture forged in *Glow* between a moving body and tracking light and images ultimately reveals itself as flawed and in the end irreconcilable. The work expresses a desire to discard or escape elements from within ourselves and this can be seen as a visual metaphor for our own constant struggle with our primitive state of duality.[26]

The strategies that allow the dancers to co-compose the performance also start to be transferred, by several art-technology collaborative groups, towards the audience. The visitors or participants can now interact with the technology and live an experience similar to the performers of the technological stage works. These technological works aim to generate a "reactive environment" or "immersive environment," a kind of "ecosystem" where the subjects are partially or totally part of the system, whether they are manipulated, following instructions, or are an important component that furthers the work's development. Although this type of active participation is not new to the arts, especially in the visual arts, there are only specific and discontinuous examples in dance.

The active participation of the audience intensifies the unpredictability, dynamism, and horizontality in stage works, emphasizing the evolving nature of the interactivity in real time. Works of dance technology with participating, immersive and/or reactive environments involve blurring the line that separates the public from the work, inviting it to experience different forms of expression and experiences of technological corporealization. The inclusion of participants who have no prior information is always a challenge, which means composing a situation that is "transparent" enough for the person visiting the environment, with instructions that enable interaction while perceiving and understanding the intention from active experience.

The latest work from the Chilean collective Emovere, *Fragile Intersections* (2019), is a performance and an installation (Instalaformance as we call it), that is a reflection on the contemporary body hybridized by the abundance of information that it experiences, modeling its subjectivity, identity and its simultaneous state between organic and artificial, between machine and flesh, sometimes individual and other times collective.[27] "Voice, sound, movement, dance, biosignals and objects converge in fragile intersections, all fused into one interactive system."[28] The immersive work consists of objects and devices that are the expression of these hybrid qualities, creating an unstable environment of sound and movement that captures the voice and biosignals of the visitors. One of these objects, Junípero, a sculpture made of paper and smart metal, responds with sinuous movements to the participants' heartbeats. On the other side of the room, Sensorium, a software, activates Junípero as it captures and processes the visitors' voices, facial features, and cardiac signals, to form a sound and visual net. The internal signals of the participants' bodies are the input for generating the installation's sound and movement; "The voice transmits the movements of the conscience, the emotion, the intent, the desire and the presence, at the same time that it has the power to communicate through language."[29]

The voice is also the basic material nature of a solo dance performance that, using the interpreter's and the public's voice, interacts with the installation's objects, as it adjusts the sound through movement sensed by the physiological sensors that capture the muscle electricity from the arms (electromyograms). So, the person who visits and participates is able to experience, wander through and relate the different elements of the instalaformance, giving his/her own body the chance to take part in the space of Fragile Intersections.

One of this work's biggest aims is to transfer the performer's own interaction and perception to the spectator, by sharing the biofeedback and self-listening that is so personal and hard to visualize in this type of interaction with physiological sensors. Therefore, the work appeals to the participants' subjectivity not only because of the different levels in which they can interrelate, but also because the material nature of their body enters into the system, as one more element that moves and transforms the space.

Undoubtedly, dance technology is a recent development that has enabled the expansion of contemporary dance. But the progress of dance technology is not progressively stable. Art with advanced technological media demands major and constant financing, since the development of new technologies requires time and the means to experiment, laboratories and specialists, as well as the dancers and choreographers willing to understand and immerse themselves in this new way of thinking about and composing dance. Generally, universities and artistic research centers with state support have usually been the place where these kinds of projects have emerged and where they have achieved some stability. Meanwhile, academic events, such as conferences, symposiums, and colloquiums are also opportunities where the exchange of specialized knowledge can generate collaborations and sustain the investigative process that this type of art needs. If the development of dance technology projects tends to be unstable in economically advanced countries, it is likely to be even more so in the economies of developing countries. However, these same countries have created projects that, working with new as well as low technologies, have taken advantage of the available possibilities.

Not only the countries that develop the most advanced technologies are suggesting the evolution of art with technology; locally developed technologies and even ancestral ones are beginning to blur the current notions of what this form of art is. We see artists and groups in emerging countries exploring new paradigms, such as low technologies and the recovery of technologies that disappeared during the conquest and colonization processes. With more access to technology the singular choreographer's vision will expand and evolve with new possibilities that are explored through software.

# FURTHER READING

Birringer, J., (ed). 2002. "Dance and Digital Media." Special issue prepared and edited for *Performing Arts Journal* 70, introduction, pp. 84–93. This paper proposes a classification on the new aesthetics of interactivity in dance, describing different types of dance interaction, depending on the technical context and the artistic challenges when working with real-time processing.

Dixon, S. 2007. *Digital Performance – A History of New Media in Theater, Dance, Performance, Art, and Installation.* The MIT Press. An excellent book that presents the historical roots, key practitioners, and artistic, theoretical, and technological trends in the incorporation of new media into the performing arts. Steve Dixon traces the evolution of these practices, presents detailed accounts of key practitioners and performances, and analyzes the theoretical, artistic, and technological contexts of this form of new media art.

Jaimovich, J. & Morand F. (2019) "Shaping the Biology of Emotion: Emovere, an Interactive Performance." *International Journal of Performance Arts and Digital Media*, 15:1, 35–52, doi:10.1080/14 794713.2018.1563354. This paper presents a detailed example of the artistic creation and research work of an interactive dance and sound performance with biosensors. *Emovere* (2015) is based on the biology of emotion in association with physiological signals and the induction of emotional states from corporeal patterns.

Wechsler, R., "Artistic Considerations in the Use of Motion Tracking with Live Performers: A Practical Guide," a chapter in the book: *Performance and Technology: Practices of Virtual Embodiment and Interactivity* edited by Susan Broadhurst and Josephine Machon, Palgrave Macmillian, 2006. This specific chapter focuses on the practical uses and the artistic implications of motion tracking, describing key concepts as interaction, real time, and mapping, as well as an analysis of one of the iconic softwares for movement interactivity: Eyecon.

# TIMELINE

Late 18th Century – Charles Louis Didelot popularizes flying machines used on stages in France.

1892 – Loïe Fuller performs "Serpentine dances."

1919–1933 – Modernism is developed, led by Rudolf Laban and the design of the Bauhaus School.

1965 – *Variations V* is performed.

1966 – Rudolf von Laban writes *Choreutics*.

1966 – "9 evenings: Theatre & Engineering" is exhibited in New York.

1980s – VNS (Very Nervous System) is created.

1990s – The term "dance technology" started to be used.

1990–1999 – LifeForms (later DanceForms) is developed and used.

2006 – *Glow* is performed.

2019 – Emovere, *Fragile Intersections* is performed.

# REFERENCES

Berringer, Johannes. (2004). "Dance and Interactivity." *Dance Research Journal* 36, 88–111.

Ceriani, Alejandra (ed) (2012). "Arte del cuerpo digital: Nuevas tecnologías y estéticas contemporáneas." Editorial de la Universidad Nacional de La Plata, Argentina.

Copeland, R. (1999). "Cunningham, Collage, and the Computer." *PAJ: A Journal of Performance and Art*, *21*(3), 42–54. https://doi.org/10.2307/3245965.

Dörr, E., & Lantz, L. (2003). "Rudolf von Laban: The 'Founding Father' of Expressionist Dance." *Dance Chronicle*, *26*(1), 1–29. Retrieved May 16, 2021, from www.jstor.org/stable/1568111.

Girão, Luís Miguel and Céu Santos, M. (2019). "The Historical Relationship between Artistic Activities and Technology Development." EPRS | European Parliamentary Research Service Scientific Foresight Unit (STOA).

Gropius, W., Wensinger, A.S., Schlemmer, O., Moholy-Nagy, L., & Molnar, F. (2014). *The Theater of the Bauhaus*. Middletown: Wesleyan University Press. muse.jhu.edu/book/36937.

Haahr, M. (2004). "The Art/Technology Interface: Innovation and Identity in Information-Age Ireland." *The Irish Review (1986-)*, (31), 40–50. doi:10.2307/29736133.

Jaimovich, J. & Morand F. (2019). "Shaping the Biology of Emotion: Emovere, an Interactive Performance." *International Journal of Performance Arts and Digital Media*, 15:1, 35–52, doi:10.1080/14794713.2018.1563354.

Lahusen, Susanne. (1986). "Oskar Schlemmer: Mechanical Ballets?" *Dance Research: The Journal of the Society for Dance Research* 4, no. 2: 65–77. Accessed August 7, 2021. doi:10.2307/1290727.

Leman, Marc. (2016). *The Expressive Moment: How Interaction (with Music) Shapes Human Empowerment*. Cambridge: The MIT Press.

McColl, Jennifer. (2012). "Bodies and Labour: Industrialisation, Dance and Performance." Thesis Master on Philosophy, School of Arts, Brunel University London.

Miller, L. (2001). "Cage, Cunningham, and Collaborators: The Odyssey of 'Variations V'." *The Musical Quarterly*, *85*(3), 545–567. Retrieved May 16, 2021, from www.jstor.org.uchile.idm. oclc.org/stable/3600996.

Moynihan, D. & Odom, L. (1984). "Oskar Schlemmer's 'Bauhaus Dances': Debra McCall's Reconstructions." *The Drama Review: TDR*, *28*(3), 46–58. doi:10.2307/1145625.

Mullis, Eric. (2013). "Dance, Interactive Technology, and the Device Paradigm." *Dance Research Journal* 46, 111–123.

Rokeby, David. (1990). "The Harmonics of Interaction." *Musicworks* 46 (Spring). Published electronically 1996. www. davidrokeby.com/harm.html.

Santana, Ivani. (2006). "Ambiguous zones: The Intertwining of Dance and World in the Technological Era." *International Journal of Performance Arts and Digital Media*, 2, 153–169

Smith, Matthew Wilson. (2007). *The Total Work of Art: From Bayreuth to Cyberspace*. Routledge, New York.

Sommer, S. (1975). "Loïe Fuller." *The Drama Review: TDR*, *19*(1), 53–67. doi:10.2307/1144969.

Swift, Mary Grace. (1974). *A Loftier Flight: The Life and Accomplishments of Charles-Louis Didelot, Balletmaster*. Wesleyan University Press. London.

Valverde, Isabel. (2012) "Interfacing Dance and Technology: Towards a Theoretical Framework for Dance in the Digital Domain." published online at cosignconference.org.

Von Bertalanffy, L. (1972). "The History and Status of General Systems Theory." *The Academy of Management Journal*, *15*(4), 407–426. doi:10.2307/255139.

Weiss, Freider. "Glow." 2006. www.frieder-weiss.de/works/all/Glow.php.

# NOTES

1. M. Haahr, (2004), "The Art/Technology Interface: Innovation and Identity in Information-Age Ireland," *The Irish Review (1986-)*, (31), 40, doi:10.2307/29736133.

2. Ivani Santana, (2006), "Ambiguous Zones: The Intertwining of Dance and World in the Technological Era," *International Journal of Performance Arts and Digital Media*, 2, 157.

3 The software Lifeforms by Credo Interactive (later Danceforms), was started by Thecla Schiphorst in 1990. www.lifeforms.com/danceforms/main.html.

4 Copeland, R. (1999), "Cunningham, Collage, and the Computer." *PAJ: A Journal of Performance and Art, 21*(3), 42–54.

5 https://dancecapsules.mercecunningham.org/overview.cfm?capid=46040.

6 www.youtube.com/watch?v=o9BiF_6gt40.

7 Santana, "Ambiguous Zones: The Intertwining of Dance and World in the Technological Era,"160.

8 Marc Leman, *The Expressive Moment: How Interaction (with Music) Shapes Human Empowerment* (Cambridge: The MIT Press: 2016), 5.

9 David Rokeby, (1990), "The Harmonics of Interaction," *Musicworks* 46 (Spring), published electronically, 1996. www.davidrokeby.com/harm.html.

10 Mary Grace Swift, *A Loftier Flight: The Life and Accomplishments of Charles-Louis Didelot, Balletmaster* (Wesleyan University Press. London, 1974), 58.

11 Swift, *A Loftier Flight*, 60

12 www.youtube.com/watch?v=Dda-BXNvVkQ.

13 Jennifer McColl, "Bodies and Labour: Industrialisation, Dance and Performance," quoted from Fuller (1913), 33–34.

14 Based on descriptions from S. Sommer.

15 Gropius, W., Wensinger, A.S., Schlemmer, O., Moholy-Nagy, L., & Molnar, F. (1986). *The Theater of the Bauhaus* (Middletown: Wesleyan University Press), 25.

16 Susanne Lahusen, "Oskar Schlemmer: Mechanical Ballets?" *Dance Research: The Journal of the Society for Dance Research* 4, no. 2: 70.

17 www.youtube.com/watch?v=-h4hOEGQRuk.

18 Matthew Wilson Smith, *The Total Work of Art: From Bayreuth to Cyberspace*. (Routledge, New York, 2007) 50.

19 https://vimeo.com/85158350.

20 www.sciencedirect.com/topics/computer-science/cybernetics.

21 McColl, "Bodies and Labour: Industrialisation, Dance and Performance," 106.

22 L. Miller, (2001), "Cage, Cunningham, and Collaborators: The Odyssey of 'Variations V'." *The Musical Quarterly, 85*(3), 561.

23 Miller, "Cage, Cunningham, and Collaborators: The Odyssey of 'Variations V'." 562.

24 www.youtube.com/watch?v=2AautwIOON8.

25 Frieder Weiss, "Glow," 2006, www.frieder-weiss.de/works/all/Glow.php.

26 Weiss, "Glow."

27 www.emovere.cl; "Intersecciones Fragiles," 2019, www.emovere.cl/intersecciones-fragiles/.

28 "Intersecciones Fragiles," 2019, www.emovere.cl/intersecciones-fragiles/.

29 "Intersecciones Fragiles," 2019, www.emovere.cl/intersecciones-fragiles/.

# CHAPTER 10

# The Future of Dance
## Moving Through Time and Space

*Monique George*

## PREDICTIONS OF TECHNOLOGICAL ADVANCEMENTS

With each new innovation in technology the immediate thought is, "What will they come up with next?" It is no secret that when we experience something new, we are already eager to explore the next big thing to be invented. There are numerous books that have predicted the evolution of technology and how it will impact how we view and interact with the world. British author H.G. Wells captured such possibilities in his scientific novels.

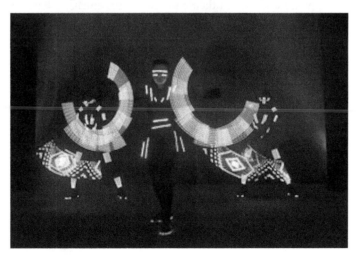

**Figure 10.1:** Dancers in LED suits with LED lamp. Photographer: Standret.

DOI: 10.4324/9781003185918-10

In his 1933 science fiction novel *The Shape of Things to Come*, Wells gives his readers a look into future events up until the year 2106. This "future history" novel tackles various issues, some of which have come to pass in real life, but also touches on how the "enlightened world citizens" in the novel are able to "breed a new race of super talents in order to maintain a permanent utopia."[1] How does this novel relate to dance in regards to advancements in technology?

## ADVANCEMENTS IN TECHNOLOGY – THE FIRST STEPS

Over time, we have witnessed technology change right before our eyes. From computers to the World Wide Web, iPads to smartphones, these are tools that have contributed to how much reach dancers, choreographers, and instructors now have. This of course could not be made possible without platforms that cater to the entertainment world as a whole. From its creation in 2005, YouTube was an early platform that paved the way for creators to post their content online, reaching a global audience. Likewise, this became a platform that dancers and choreographers use to upload their works and expand their audiences exponentially. Now, 16 years later, YouTube has evolved into a virtual video tool for dancers to not only showcase their works but to also post instructional videos that reach millions of dancers around the world. So, for someone who lives in New Zealand or Japan, a lesson in the *Graham* or *Horton* techniques is now within arm's reach.

YouTube was a technological innovation that started an access phenomenon in how companies and choreographers could reach not only live audiences but also asynchronous audiences around the world. Instagram was the next vessel of social media that aimed to build upon how people shared their content and communicated with one another. While gaining momentum almost instantaneously due to its growth in popularity, Instagram has proven to be another platform that artists use to their advantage. How would Instagram and Instagram Live revolutionize how we perceive various forms of dance? More importantly, what could this do for instructors around the world wanting to share their knowledge and expertise? This is where advancements in technology would meet education in a blissful union – a seemingly attainable goal, but also with inherent challenges.

## TECHNOLOGY AND DANCE EDUCATION – THE GREAT MERGER?

It is no surprise that technology has changed how we search for, find, and in return, take in information. We have almost gone from having to be physically present to learn to now being able to remotely open the doors of knowledge from the comfort of our own homes. How each individual learns is not created equal, but the accelerated rate by which technology is evolving has thrust educators to adjust how they reach their students. Zihao Li's article, "Mobile technology in dance education," sheds light on the pros and cons that technological advances can impact the lens through which we view dance education. For a dance pedagogy, could technology serve as a catalyst for our current climate while also effectively altering how we approach learning?

Li does not deny that technology offers certain allowances for dance teaching to enter into new territories, however, he does point out where initial issues come into play before the benefits can be recognized. Noting the challenges in the current state of dance education, Li points out,

> 'Research shows that technology is generally used as an isolated product disconnected from classroom instruction (Crystal, 2006). The use of technology in dance education appears to be more limited than other disciplines.' When we think of mastering dance, more importantly the technique that comes with it, one must also keep in mind that even today not everyone may have access to technological resources outside of what they've learned in class.[2]

(Li, 2011)

Li offers the plausible scenario of an instructor that teaches a fusion of *Limon* and *Graham* techniques, but the availability of resources for this type of fusion are extremely limited online. Though he concludes that the results of the scenario are not promising, there is the undeniable recognition that, when used with the right goal in mind and openness to change, technology can serve a bigger purpose in a high-speed environment. Even so, one must wonder if it is plausible for dance educators to reach their students adequately through **cyberspace**. Can technology advancement both serve the students of various backgrounds and also the educator involved?

Today we live in a "cyber generation" especially when it comes to young teens and adults. We have graduated from accessing what we want strictly from our in-person experiences and our TVs to having instant access to programing in the palm of our hands. This has become a game changer for reaching technology savvy students and widening the way we approach dance curriculum as a whole. While dance used to be seen as something that could only be taught in a studio, library space, or even a gym, it has become more relevant for dance educators to find more efficient ways to reach larger numbers of students through advancements in technology. By establishing a "hub" of sorts for students to access materials and communicate with their instructors, dance education has taken a hybrid approach which has broken the stigma associated with where and when dancers can learn and enjoy a class.

As he explored and surveyed the implementation of technology in dance education at York University while teaching modern and ballet technique between 2009 and 2010, Li investigated the potential of using technology in his teaching by creating a multimedia website. This multimedia site consisted of general course information like PDF forms for course outlines and assignments, interactive blogs, and podcasts that monitored the physical and mental progress of dance students. The end goal was to see how this implementation of technology could meaningfully enhance dance teaching and learning.

There are pros and cons with introducing new approaches and techniques which can apply to most situations. With regard to enhancing the dance education experience, this survey in particular served as a catalyst to what could be done better and what worked overall for the participants involved. The pros outweighed the cons while opening up more opportunity for the students involved to find a middle ground between in-person learning and virtual learning. Flexibility is one of the key factors that comes into play when one has to determine how technology will benefit or hinder the educational process. More often than not, especially in areas of higher education, it is beneficial for a student who has a heavy workload to know that they can come back to a lesson they have missed without fear of falling behind. The same can be said for dancers who have to keep up with their technique while also balancing other commitments.

Li points out that with the advancement of technology and an ever-growing online community,

> dance education has entered into a new era. As dance educators, we have to maintain our focus. As Hong, Caldwell, Ashley & Alpert (2009) suggest, we need to 're-examine, re-consider and re-tool our pedagogical paradigms and practices. We must constantly remind ourselves that it is our activity as reflective artists, administrators, and educators engaged in the pursuit and provision of scholarly teaching and research that enlarges and advances learning within and across discipline fields.'[3]

Even with the advantages that Li witnessed through the York University survey, he notes that dance educators must still keep in mind that "while using technology to improve pedagogical approaches, technology is merely an enhancement and cannot substitute for content that promotes learning and critical thinking within and across subject areas."[4] Though he concludes that the *physical* aspect of dance training can "never be replaced" by the advancement of technology, what can be said for when there is no choice but to train virtually? Is it actually possible for dancers to grow physically through virtual learning? In the future will educators still reach said dancers through advancements in technology alone?

## SOCIAL MEDIA, LIVESTREAMING, AND INSTRUCTIONAL VIDEOS

Twenty years ago, the thought of someone being able to take consistent dance technique classes let alone a master class virtually would have been unheard of. Just as technology was evolving, the art of dance was following suit, which began to bridge the gap that stood between dance education and technology. Virtual instruction came to us in the form of video tapes and televised programing but took a swift jump when online platforms became available. As mentioned before, YouTube was somewhat of a pioneer in the way dancers could absorb educational materials apart from their studio setting. Imagine being able to further your craft with various instructors all over the world from the comfort of a computer. To take it even further, imagine being able to take these materials around with you in the palm of your hand (i.e., tablet or smartphone). It couldn't get better than that, right?

Apart from being able to post instructional videos for dancers of all nationalities to utilize, there was yet another revolutionary concept that would further jolt the way dance educators could reach their students – **livestreaming**. This proved to be a game changer for industries across the board, but more importantly the dance community. Imagine living in the United Kingdom and being able to take a master class with *Royal Family Dance Crew* from Auckland, New Zealand without having to catch a flight. For those who wanted to take a modern class at the Alvin Ailey School, it was now possible through live streaming globally without having to travel to New York City. There was now a door to real-time interaction even if students couldn't physically be there in person. Social platforms such as Facebook and Instagram wasted no time introducing the livestreaming experience as well. Dancers and choreographers alike had yet another technological tool at their disposal.

Competitive dance in particular has taken the livestream experience by storm. As dance competitions tour various countries, it is evident that spectators and commentators cannot realistically travel to every event. For the competitive dance circuit, livestreaming has taken advantage of that need for real-time experience by catering their platforms to make it seem like spectators and competitors are in the same auditorium. Regional and national competitions have now made their events accessible to anyone with a smartphone, tablet, or computer that wants to share the same excitement that they may have missed out on otherwise. In the light of COVID-19 and safety concerns, the competitive circuit is now starting to see virtual competitions and conventions popping up. How will this new approach to competitive dance contribute to how we experience competition dance in the future?

Currently, though virtual competitions are few and far between, the popularity of this new approach to competitive dance has not gone unnoticed. One of the main benefits with virtual dance competitions is the way they utilize various social media platforms to generate traffic and create buzz. Dance companies from all over the world now compete virtually in a variety of dance genres. Imagine being able to enter a Bollywood dance routine from Mumbai and compete with a traditional Chinese dance routine from Beijing. What an amazing way for two different dance worlds to engage with one another and enjoy a dance style that they may not have been exposed to before. Virtual dance competitions not only open a new door to how dancers experience competition, but also to rewarding opportunities for the judges involved as well. Expectations are shifted not only because of greater reach but there is also an element of the unexpected. This differs quite a bit from what judges have experienced in person in the not-so-distant past especially with local competitions. Furthermore, this can alleviate any preconceived biases based on the dance companies entering.

Like any new venture, there are still some traditional aspects that align with the "normal" competition experience. There are specific divisions which dance companies can enter based on skill level as well as a variety of dance genres they can choose to compete in. Having it all fall under a virtual platform lightens the load of processing entries and award categories because they now fall under one big hub. Though there isn't the build-up of excitement that one would experience competing in person, dancers, choreographers, and special awards can still be recognized virtually. While it may not be everyone's go-to, virtual dance competitions still afford a platform for young dancers to showcase their talent and get viable feedback while keeping themselves and others safe during moments of health crisis such as a pandemic. Some may say that's a win-win, but this does not take away from an individual's need for one-on-one training and feedback. Is it *truly* possible to continue training on a virtual platform and still feel like you're in class?

## ZOOM DANCE CLASSES, VIRTUAL REALITY, AND VIRTUAL WORLDS – THE MIDDLEMAN

As people, we crave human-to human contact – even more so as artists. It's in our DNA. Whether we admit it or not, there is something about encountering a person or merely being around them that helps us grow or simply get through the day. We've discussed the great debate of technology being able to truly serve as a co-pilot to teachers and choreographers in dance education. Though there have been years spent being conditioned to being trained in a studio with hands-on critiquing from instructors, the mindset has had to evolve over time with technological innovation. While livestreaming and instructional videos serve as great supplementary materials for dancers to enhance how they absorb every technique thrown their way, the missing link is actual physical contact. Keeping safety in mind, how could someone further their training in a highly technical style such as ballet or modern at home while still getting much needed attention to detail?

In the future, teaching class would almost seem impossible to conduct completely virtually especially for those who know how much work goes into in-person learning. After all, dance has historically been a field of mentorship. Even so, when there are too many risks involved (i.e., a pandemic or weather-related closure) there would seem to be no other choice but to cancel class. However, that is not the case anymore thanks to yet another innovation; Zoom. Although created over a decade ago in 2011, the idea of using Zoom would have been an afterthought for choreographers and dance educators, but when businesses were forced to close due to COVID-19 there had to be a way to keep motivation alive as well as routine. This was no different for studio owners striving to keep the dance season going as safely as possible and keeping dancers trained except to embrace Zoom. Although it was met with initial hesitation, the common denominator for studios across the globe is Zoom now.

This platform like many others is not void of any faults as far as connection issues or minor glitches, but more often than not it offered dance studios and companies an opportunity to conduct live classes in order to keep momentum going even if it meant doing so from a living room or basement. Dance educators were forced to reprogram their approach to technique classes. What this sudden shift did was force dancers to be even more aware of their bodies while adjusting to the unconventional spaces they designated as their studios. Taking classes through Zoom also forced instructors to figure out how they could correct students without physical contact. While it would seem that this was more of a hindrance than helpful at first, what most found is that they could closely pinpoint exactly where they could improve their technique by relying on self-sufficiency to make said corrections since their instructors were not able to fix them as they would in a normal class setting. More so, being in front of a screen while following a teacher on the other side also forced dancers to critically think in regard to what direction they needed to be moving in a combination or whether they should be mirroring what they saw.

Although studios have slowly created efficient safety protocols for in-person learning that dancers and teachers have to follow to keep studio spaces safe and workable, there is still the possibility that Zoom may be the go-to in the event of a severe weather closure or even another pandemic. It may also be, in such instances, the platform that keeps a recital or company performance from being canceled. With this in mind, what could this mean for professional dance companies? How has this shift in how classes have been taught translate to how we may experience performances in the future? Though Zoom may seem to be the only viable solution and the closest to live interaction and performance, virtual reality may take the realistic experience to new heights.

Even as a topic of the early 1900s, virtual reality is still a concept that is fairly new to our world of ever-growing technology. It has been a staple in the gaming community with growing popularity for those who want to be "fully immersed" in the action. Imagine being able to fight in a full contact ring or dodging zombies in another with a simple headset. Now switch these scenarios to being a dancer on the stage of the Sydney Opera House and you've opened up a world of possibilities that could innovate an entire artistic movement. It would be a captivating experience to jump into a modern dance class and actually see the marley dance floor beneath your feet and the mirrors surrounding you in the studio. To go a step further, imagine seeing and feeling the presence of other students and experiencing the instructor in the same space giving feedback. This may have seemed far-fetched 20 years ago, but could this be an innovation that dancers, choreographers, and teachers may make use of more as we discover more ways to ignite and spark passion for artistry?

"Virtual Reality and Choreographic Practice: The Potential for New Creative Methods" ventures into the many possibilities virtual reality presents for dancers and choreographers.[5] As virtual reality (VR) becomes a more enticing arena for dancers and choreographers, it is sparking an even greater incentive for creators to develop the necessary tools to make this dream a reality. As noted in Chapter 9, VR is an immersive technology that, when used in performance, is an instrument for co-creation between the audience, dancers,

and choreographers. It can also be used to enhance learning. WhoLoDancE: Whole-Body Interaction Learning for
Dance Education is in the development stages for tools that
will allow virtual reality and dance education to intersect.
With an interdisciplinary team including dancers, choreographers, educators, artists, coders, technologists, and system
architects, the early stages of testing and working with end-
users has helped with gathering thoughts about the issues
that could emerge in the creation of said tools.[6] According
to VR expert Koster, "a virtual world is a spatially based
depiction of a persistent virtual environment, which can be
experienced by numerous participants at once, who are represented within the space by avatars."[7] What does this say
when focusing on the dancer who is directly experiencing
the virtual world?

When exploring virtual reality and its impact on the field, it
is important to note the individual's knowledge of the tools
used to make the ultimate experience possible. The focus of
the WhoLoDancE project is to explore ways in which the
"virtual environment can augment and contribute to dance
learning and expand choreographic techniques."[8] Keeping
this in mind, one must assume that the dancer will be able
to fully immerse themselves in the technology being used,
but in order to do so it will take much more understanding of the tools associated with optimizing the virtual reality
experience. Integrating expensive and technically demanding equipment is not always possible, so this is where the
WhoLoDancE project has had to navigate the challenges
that would come throughout the planning and experimental
stages.

It is important to note that one of the intentions mentioned
with the use of virtual reality technologies is to create new
kinds of immersive experiences that offer the dancer a chance
to learn independently with a virtual teacher by being able
to dance with a dance expert or even the dancer's own
projected image. Keeping this in mind, one of the many
challenges to be conquered was offering the choreographers
and dance students tools that would be meaningful, accessible, useful, intuitive. These would not only contribute to

advancing the field of dance but also support the needs of dance artists, teachers, and learners alike. So, are these new technologies set out to completely replace the live experience that dancers have become accustomed to? And if so, will this work to benefit all who are involved?

Ultimately, there is no way to fully replace the live experience that dancers and choreographers have known and depend on for the spirit of growth. However, the approach taken by WhoLoDancE speaks volumes to future-looking learning styles by developing tools that don't set out to enhance and expand current practices that are used on a normal basis and push the boundaries of the dance art form rather than replacing the live experience or teacher altogether. There are still quite a few factors that need to be taken into consideration. The WhoLoDancE project was proactive in taking into account variety in their approach not only with the VR tools that were presented but what dance genres could serve as guinea pigs so to speak. Greek folk, ballet, contemporary, and flamenco were just some of the dance genres that the project focused on with attention to the terminology used in each genre as well.

While collaborating with partners from the dance community, a dialogic process which kept specific requirements in mind for the design of tools to make the VR experiment a reality began to take shape. According to Cisneros, Wood, Whatley, Buccoli, Zanoni, and Sarti, the tools that are essential for the WhoLoDancE project to venture into success have been tested in several demonstration events in various European countries including the U.K. in an effort to collect feedback for improving usability. Usability is a key player in the game of VR merging with the dance community. Factors such as accessibility and usability with technology only scratch the surface when we take into account how having a headset on could significantly alter the user's mode of balance or spatial awareness. For those involved in the creating process for the WhoLoDancE project, new ventures like dancing in a motion capture studio, wearing tight suits with optical markers, and performing in a studio surrounded by cameras were explored.

These highly technical attributes, along with special software, works as one to compute 3D space as well as 3D positions and orientation of the dancers such as their head, spine, arms, and legs. For WhoLoDancE, the focus steadied on the smaller gestures and movements for each particular genre as it was motion captured such as a hand or finger movement in flamenco dance. With a way to record movements under their belt, that could not be the end of exploration into VR technology recreating dance techniques. What happens for those who want to revisit said movements from particular genres such as ballet, flamenco, or Greek folk dance? The answer came in the form of the *Movement Library*.[9] The *Movement Library* allows users to annotate each recording with qualities, properties, or actions through an easy-to-use interface and those annotations are then used to retrieve items in the library.

In addition to the *Movement Library*, *Sketching* tools are also useful because they provide dance students and choreographers with examples of movements. The set of movements also lend themselves to "research scenarios as they can enable researchers to investigate similarities among *steps* across different genres."[10] While we have focused mainly on the education portion of dance and channeling the technical movements by means of VR, where does the choreographic element fit into this scenario? Through a choreographic tool known as the *Blending Engine*, the users can mix and match different movements, and build an avatar that could perform several combinations of "steps" and movement phrases. The upside for choreographers who have access to the *Blending Engine* is the ability to use "search by similarity and by movement" sketching to retrieve recordings from the *Movement Library* and essentially combine them to make a whole new performance.

This phenomenon has been an inspiration for choreographers thus far and has sparked a revolutionary movement of how audiences receive choreography from a virtual standpoint. Visualization and realism can be expressed in avatar form and with that comes curiosity as to how we know and experience dance performance and how different our experience would be along with audiences from across the world. The article "Is Virtual Reality the Future of Dance?" by Carla Escoda tackles the performance aspect of dance as an artform and how impactful the possibilities could be when including VR in the performance realm. Escoda touches on how VR was solely limited to gamers, adventure seekers, and simulation builders is now something of the past and that it may surprise patrons to see how dance-makers have employed this technology on screen.[11] In 2017, the San Francisco Dance Film Festival put this idea to the test when they screened a handful of 360° and VR dance films at San Francisco's Brava Theater in the hopes of grabbing viewer's attention and ultimately pulling them into another world.

It would have been expected that these types of films would have been met with skepticism and maybe a bit of unrest knowing they would be viewed with a machine strapped to people's heads. Even so, as Escoda explains it, "no film can replicate the thrill of live dance of the dancer's sense of precariousness."[12] *Through You* (2017) was one of the films shown at the San Francisco Dance Film Festival that set out to bring the authentic feeling of a live performance under the team of film director Saschka Unseld in addition to director and choreographer Lily Baldwin. According to Escoda, the pair sought to create an authentic sense of place and a palpable connection to the dancers by shooting on location. The beauty of *Through You* was caught with about 200 cuts which was a huge contrast to the normal VR filmmaking process, which afforded the film a dream-like quality.[13] From the outside looking in, the viewer was teleported into each scene and the emotion that the dancers exuded in some instances evoked immense feelings from the viewer in return. How could these VR experiences, experienced through the San Francisco Dance Film Festival, shape how we experience dance performances while still connecting with the performers on a more emotional level?

The beauty of dance films, especially those that incorporate VR is that they can whisk viewers away from the real world and transport you into unimaginable settings that would only otherwise be experienced in dreams. As Escoda points out, "Even when there are no human dancers visible on screen, viewer disembodiment can amplify a mood." Cecilia Sweet-Coll's film *Anicca* (2016) is a prime example of disembodiment in which the motion captured from dancers animates a mysterious and whimsical landscape.[14] The spirit of fully immersing viewers has also given way to films that seek to put viewers in the center of an unfolding tradition, rather than create a sense of disembodiment like works such as *A History of Cuban Dance* (2016) and the *Paul Taylor Dance Company 360° Brochure* (2017). Both of these works offered viewers a unique perspective on the evolution of a body of work. In her experience, Escoda had a firsthand adventure of sorts wandering around a virtual recreation of Cuba with a VR headset on which afforded her a powerful sensation of the live experience of dance. The barriers that most would experience between dancers, musicians, and audience were non-existent and created a performance space for viewers to be a part of as well.

Perspective is one of the main things that one must consider when tackling the question – can audiences adequately experience a dance performance through VR with the feeling of being seated in a theater? Because of the importance of grabbing the audience's attention and portraying the story of each number, it is essential that this emotion translates from each dancer's body through the lens that thousands of eyes will get to experience. The upside of the phenomenon that comes from these experiences is that the performers, orchestra, and scenery are no longer separate entities but one immersive unit with endless possibilities. There are, and will continue to be, improvements that must be made from a technological as well as an economic standpoint, but the interest in seeing how VR can play a pivotal role in immersive experience and site-specific dance has not been deterred so far. Growing interest in these avenues will not seek to replace the traditional live dance experiences for patrons but rather widen the spectrum of dance performance as a whole, thus granting companies to reach global audiences while widening their digital footprint.

# ROBOTS AND HOLOGRAMS – THE NEW FRONTIER

What other frontiers are left to explore for performance experiences and enrichment? There cannot be one specific answer to this question, but one thing is certain; the possibilities have become endless as people discover more innovative ways to keep the artform alive. One example that sparks this notion of where dance's future may be headed was seen in 2014 on the Billboard Music Awards stage. The death of Michael Jackson in 2009 was one that shook not only the music industry but fans of his music and iconic dance moves. No one could have imagined seeing the "King of Pop" perform again, but with nearly half a year of planning prior to the 2014 Billboard Music Awards, which included filming, choreography, and the development of new technology, the showstopping performance under the sleeves of producers was in holographic form.

Not only was there a special stage built specifically for the holographic performance along with 16 additional dancers live on stage to "Slave to the Rhythm," but the **hologram** of Jackson dancing signature routines that became a staple to his artistry including the moonwalk was the icing on the cake. Looking back at that performance, one must wonder what this could mean for touring artists or even companies showcasing their works cross country or even overseas. Holograms seem to be the most "life-like" experiences because of the way they can capture the body's movements as well as the little nuances in facial expressions. Holograms are quite literally a snapshot with assistance from a lens and give the illusion that the artist or dancer is right on stage or any other arena. For touring dance companies this could be beyond revolutionary because it affords the chance for repertory works to be performed as it is envisioned by the choreographer but in multiple locations at the same time. Imagine experiencing a performance from The Royal Ballet in Los Angeles in holographic form while there are simultaneous performances happening in New York or even Wellington. This would be impossible for live dancers but with the technology of holograms, it would broaden the reach to multiple audiences while keeping their repertoire true to form.

The same could be said for choreographers wanting to workshop classes and optimize the number of dancers they may impact. Being able to teach multiple dancers across many locations would have been unfathomable up until recently. Now there is more room for the impossible with the help of technology and the need to keep experiences as authentic as humanly possible. How amazing would it be to take class from the great legends like the late Alvin Ailey or Bob Fosse through the means of holograms? Much like the experience that millions witnessed on the Billboard Music Awards stage in 2014, it is safe to predict that holograms will soon be a norm in our technological age and with teams of artists and scientists working towards making this happen, audiences will get to experience performances in ways they never could have imagined.

Apart from holograms, robots are another form of evolving technology that comes to mind when thinking of where dance, dance education, and choreography can advance and ultimately grow. Just as dancers learn techniques consistent with the genre of dance they're focused on, robots are programed in certain ways through computer technology to perform various tasks. Can the two go hand in hand when it comes to robots and dance? To go a step further, is it possible for a robot to be programed to choreograph a dance or teach? Though it is more than possible for a robot to "dance" in many respects, one reservation that may come up is if said movement can be aesthetically pleasing to the eye. Though there is very little range of motion, most of which is sharp or staccato, there is still room for speculation that robots could have a place in dance performance. After all, there are choreographic works like those of Alwin Nikolais that are based on "dehumanized dance" where dancers move in a mechanical way similar to what one would expect from a robot. So, it is safe to assume that it is possible for a robot to be programed to teach or even choreograph for human dancers even if it is unconventional to the traditional approach that most are used to.

245

# THE FUTURE OF DANCE MOVING FORWARD

Revisiting safety concerns and our ever-changing world, the biggest question is where does dance go from here? Will the new norm be dependent solely on the integration of technology along with dance? In addition to the unknown, is it possible that dance as an artform will migrate to different arenas besides theaters? Just like astronauts continue to explore life on other planets like Mars, it may not be too far-fetched that we will be able to bring dance performances to other planets which would provide a visual and experience never seen before. We have only scratched the surface of how dance has evolved and will continue to do so as we soar to technological heights. The world quite literally can become a stage for choreographers to challenge themselves and for dancers to utilize. We could possibly use the ocean as a new arena to explore choreographic works and widen the imagination of viewers and see what impact it has on dancers as well. Will we be exposed to forms of time travel that make it possible for touring companies to perform in London or France and be able to take a high-speed train or flight to California to perform for another set of audiences? Where do we go next? What do *you* envision for the future of dance?

## FURTHER READING

Bleeker, Maaike. "Transmission in Motion: The Technologizing of Dance."1st Edition. ISBN 9781138189447. October 4, 2016 by Routledge. When we discuss motion, more specifically dance, there is a personalization and realism that we expect. There is a need to feel and see things from a human perspective that we may not expect to be attainable through technology. However, "Transmission in Motion: The Technologizing of Dance" strives to show the mutual connection between various technologies, from a conventional standpoint to newer avenues, and how those can be used to better understand dance movement.

Dixon, Steve. "Digital Performance: A History of New Media in Theater, Dance, Performance Art, and Installation" ISBN: 9780262042352828 pp. | 7 in. x 9 in. 235 illus. February 2007. New technology takes time to fine tune as people experiment with better modes of functionality. Over the past decade, we have seen an emergence of technology combined with the arts. In this digital age that we live in, there are more possibilities in how audiences can fully experience performances even if it is not in the traditional "live" arena. Dixon explores the changes in how body, time, and space are represented while acknowledging newer technologies such as avatars, virtual bodies, and digital doubles.

Sparshott, Francis. "The Future of Dance Aesthetics." *The Journal of Aesthetics and Art Criticism* 51, no. 2 (1993): 227–234. doi:10.2307/431389. Aesthetics plays a pivotal role in how we perceive things around us. This pertains to many aspects of life whether scientific, philosophical, etc. The arts is no different when it comes to aesthetics, which begs the question of how the subject of aesthetics could coincide with technology and how it relates to the future of where dance will go.

Tharp, T. "On Technology and Dance." *Encyclopedia Britannica*, July 22, 2005. www.britannica.com/topic/technology-and-dance-1082484. How technology can contribute to dance and the way we view dance education and performance is a question with many possible answers. Tharp dives into the ways which we have come accustomed to receiving dance performance while highlighting how technology elevates that experience.

## TIMELINE

February 14, 2005 – Youtube is launched.

October 6, 2010 – Instagram is launched.

2014 – A hologram of Michael Jackson is screened at the Billboard Music Awards stage.

2017 – *Through You* is released.

2019 – WhoLoDancE project begins.

March 2020 – COVID-19 prompts series of lockdowns.

## BIBLIOGRAPHY

Bell, Mark W. "Toward a Definition of 'Virtual Worlds'." *The Journal of Virtual Worlds Research* 1 (2008): 1.

Cisneros, R.E., Wood, K., Whatley, S., Buccoli, M., Zanoni, M., and Sarti, A. (2019). "Virtual Reality and Choreographic Practice: The Potential for New Creative Methods." *Body, Space*

& *Technology*, 18(1), pp. 1–32. DOI: http://doi.org/10.16995/bst.305.

Escoda, Carla. (Oct. 16, 2017). "Is Virtual Reality the Future of Dance?" www.kqed.org/arts/13811546/is-virtual-reality-the-future-of-dance.

Gray, Judith A. Ed. (1989). "Dance Technology: Current Applications and Future Trends."

Wells, H.G. (1895). "The Time Machine."

Zihao Li, Mingming Zhou, and Timothy Teo. (2018). "Mobile Technology in Dance Education: A Case Study of Three Canadian High School Dance Programs." *Research in Dance Education* 19:2, pp. 183–196.

# NOTES

1 H.G. Wells. (1895). "The Time Machine."

2 Zihao Li, Mingming Zhou, and Timothy Teo (2018). "Mobile Technology in Dance Education: A Case Study of Three Canadian High School Dance Programs," *Research in Dance Education* 19:2, 183–196.

3 Li, "Mobile Technology in Dance Education: A Case Study of Three Canadian High School Dance Programs," 12.

4 Li, "Mobile Technology in Dance Education: A Case Study of Three Canadian High School Dance Programs," 12.

5 R.E. Cisneros, Wood, K., Whatley, S., Buccoli, M., Zanoni, M., and Sarti, A. (2019). "Virtual Reality and Choreographic Practice: The Potential for New Creative Methods," *Body, Space & Technology*, 18(1), 1–32. DOI: http://doi.org/10.16995/bst.305.

6 Cisneros, "Virtual Reality and Choreographic Practice: The Potential for New Creative Methods."

7 Mark W. Bell, "Toward a Definition of 'Virtual Worlds'," *The Journal of Virtual Worlds Research* 1 (2008): 1.

8 Cisneros, "Virtual Reality and Choreographic Practice: The Potential for New Creative Methods."

9 Cisneros, "Virtual Reality and Choreographic Practice: The Potential for New Creative Methods."

10 Cisneros, "Virtual Reality and Choreographic Practice: The Potential for New Creative Methods."

11 Carla Escoda (Oct. 16, 2017). "Is Virtual Reality the Future of Dance?" www.kqed.org/arts/13811546/is-virtual-reality-the-future-of-dance.s

12 Escoda, "Is Virtual Reality the Future of Dance?"

13 Escoda, "Is Virtual Reality the Future of Dance?"

14 Escoda, "Is Virtual Reality the Future of Dance?"

# Timeline

500–800 CE – Sogdian trade with China peaks, trading luxuries, such as gemstones, horses, grape wine, precious metals, amber, furs, slaves, and foreign dancers. (Chapter 2)

755–763 CE – Rebellion of the General An Lushan results in foreigners and foreign ideas becoming regarded with suspicion. (Chapter 2)

1200s – Māori ancestors settle in Aotearoa. (Chapter 5)

Late 1300s–1400s – Ballet is created in Italy. (Chapter 4)

1525 – Middle Passage begins. For the next 300-plus years, Portuguese, Dutch, British, French, Spanish, and other European nations enslave Africans and transport them to the Western Hemisphere. (Chapter 3)

1526–1858 – The Mughal Dynasty values poets, architects, painters, musicians, craftsmen, religious scholars, and dancers. (Chapter 2)

1533 – Catherine de Medici moves to France, bringing ballet de cour or ballet of the court. (Chapter 4)

16th–19th century – Enslaved Africans in the Western Hemisphere continue dance traditions from their homelands and develop new ones. Religious practices that incorporate dance include Vodou in Haiti, Santería in Cuba, Candomblé in Brazil, Hoodoo in Louisiana, and Obeah throughout the Caribbean. Martial art dance forms, such as capoeira in Brazil and ladja/danmyé in Martinique, also develop, as well as countless social dances, such as the Cakewalk in the Southern United States and tango in Argentina. (Chapter 3)

1608 – British arrive in India. (Chapter 2)

1642 – Dutch explorers land in Aotearoa. (Chapter 5)

1661 – Louis XIV forms the Académie Royale de Danse, the first state funded school for ballet. (Chapter 4)

1689 – Ballet reaches Moscow. (Chapter 4)

Late 18th Century – Charles Louis Didelot popularizes flying machines used on stages in France. (Chapter 9)

1776 – The Bolshoi Ballet is founded. (Chapter 4)

Early 1800s – Romantic era of ballet begins, with notable performances such as *Giselle*. (Chapter 4)

1800s – Dance and mindful movement as a process for healing begins to be articulated by performing artists such as Èmile Jacques-Dalcroze and François Delsarte. (Chapter 7)

1840s – William Henry Lane, or "Master Juba," showcases his innovative blend of West African aesthetics and Irish jigging to become one of the most famous stage performers in the world. Countless white men in blackface imitate him in the new theatrical genre of minstrelsy, which develops in the United States. Lane's dance aesthetics become influential in the development of tap, jazz, and step dancing. (Chapter 3)

1857 – The British Crown seizes control of India. (Chapter 2)

1860s–1880s – Black US Americans replace white performers in minstrel shows, further innovating and refining Black social dances for the theatrical stage. (Chapter 3)

1876 – Battle of Greasy Grass occurs, when Lakota people, along with the Northern Cheyenne and Arapaho, defeat the 7th Cavalry Regiment. (Chapter 1)

1890 – Wounded Knee Massacre. (Chapter 1)

1890s–1910s – In the United States, Aida Overton Walker and other Black US American choreographers transition from minstrelsy to vaudeville, shedding blackface and caricatured stereotypes to promote revised performances of the Cakewalk and other ragtime dances. (Chapter 3)

1892 – Loïe Fuller performs "Serpentine dances." (Chapter 9)

1892 or 1893 – Michio Itō is born in Tokyo, Japan. (Chapter 6)

1896 – Film is first presented in India at Watson's Hotel in Bombay. (Chapter 8)

1904 – Loie Fuller released her first film. (Chapter 8)

1909 – Serge Diaghilev forms the Ballets Russes. (Chapter 4)

1910 – Cinema halls are built in every major Indian city. (Chapter 8)

1913 – India's first film, *Raja Harischandra*, is released. (Chapter 8)

1914 – Japan declares war on Germany; Itō moves to England. (Chapter 6)

1915 – Edgar John Rubin conceptualizes Rubin's Vase. (Chapter 5)

1915–1934 – US occupies Haiti. (Chapter 3)

1916 – *The Dumb Girl of Portici* featuring Anna Pavlova is released. (Chapter 8)

1916 – Itō creates his signature solo, *Pizzacati*. (Chapter 6)

1917 – *The Dying Swan* featuring Anna Pavlova is released. (Chapter 8)

1919–1933 – Modernism is developed, led by Rudolf Laban and the design of the Bauhaus School. (Chapter 9)

1920s – Busby Berkeley choreographs for numerous Broadway musicals. (Chapter 8)

1920s – The international New Negro Movement promotes the celebration of African cultural roots and asserts a new political consciousness in challenging white supremacy, colonialism, and imperialism. Martinican Aimé Cesaire coins the term *negritude*, roughly understood as a Black consciousness. In Cuba, there is the Afro-Cubanismo movement; in Haiti, the indigenisme movement; in the United States, the Harlem Renaissance. Africanist dance aesthetics become central to stage performances across the Americas. On Broadway, tap and jazz dominate. (Chapter 3)

1921 – Tulsa Race Massacre: a violent white mob kills hundreds of people and destroys the Greenwood District, also known as America's Black Wall Street. (Chapter 5)

1924 – The Immigration Act of 1924 limits the number of allowed immigrants to the United States. (Chapter 5)

1928–1929 – Itō's company goes on tour. (Chapter 6)

1929 – Itō stages *The New World Symphony*. (Chapter 6)

1930s – Katherine Dunham and Zora Neale Hurston, Black US Americans, conduct ethnographic research in the Caribbean and document many dance forms, including the shay-shay in Jamaica, the mazouk in Martinique, and the beguine in Haiti. Dunham begins to incorporate these dances into her choreography, performed on Broadway and on stages across the globe. (Chapter 3)

1931 – Alam Ara ("The Beauty of the World"), the first Indian film with full sound, is released. (Chapter 8)

1933 – Berkeley becomes the dance director of *The Gold Diggers of 1933*. (Chapter 8)

1933 – Fred Astaire makes his film debut in *Dancing Lady*. (Chapter 8)

1934 – George Balanchine and Lincoln Kirstein found American Ballet, now called the School of American Ballet (SAB). (Chapter 4)

1939 – American Ballet Theatre (ABT) is founded by Lucia Chase, Richard Pleasant, and Oliver Smith in New York City. (Chapter 4)

1940 – Laura Perls co-creates Gestalt Therapy. (Chapter 7)

1940–1960 – Dancers teach in hospitals, schools for the deaf, differently abled children, orphanages, and other institutions. (Chapter 7)

1940s–1960s – Across the Americas, national dance troupes are formed that highlight and promote Africanist aesthetics, including the National Dance Theatre Company of Jamaica, founded by Rex Nettleford. Individuals such as Jean-Leon Destiné of Haiti and Alvin Ailey in the United States form their own companies, not necessarily tied to a national identity, and tour the world. Afro-Caribbean social dances such as mambo, rhumba, and calypso become the rage across the Americas. (Chapter 3)

1941 – December 7 – The Japanese attack Pearl Harbor. (Chapter 6)

1941 – December 8 – The U.S. government arrests Itō. (Chapter 6)

1942 – February 19 – President Franklin D. Roosevelt signs Executive Order 9066. (Chapter 6)

1942 – April – Itō is moved between internment camps at Fort Sill in Oklahoma, and then to Camp Livingston in Louisiana. (Chapter 6)

1943 – Michio Itō repatriates to Japan. (Chapter 6)

1944 – *Appalachian Spring* is performed. (Chapter 5)

1944 – Gene Kelly directs "Alter Ego" in *Cover Girl*. (Chapter 8)

1950s – Mary Starks Whitehouse develops "Authentic Movement." (Chapter 7)

1954 – January 26 – Dancers represent PEPSU to perform for the Republic Day festivities in New Delhi. (Chapter 2)

1955 – Arthur Mitchell joins New York City Ballet. (Chapter 4)

1960s – The Black Arts Movement emerges in the United States, which reaffirms the social and political consciousness of Black art and the need to turn to Africa, instead of Europe, for aesthetic principles and practices. West African music and dance classes become a part of dance studios, community centers, and higher education curricula. (Chapter 3)

1961 – Jerome Robbins directs *West Side Story*. (Chapter 8)

1961 – Michio Itō dies in Tokyo. (Chapter 6)

1965 – Malcolm X is assassinated. (Chapter 5)

1965 – U.S. immigration law abolishes de facto discrimination against Asians, causing many Punjabis to move to the U.S. (Chapter 2)

1965 – *Variations V* is performed. (Chapter 9)

1966 – "9 evenings: Theatre & Engineering" is exhibited in New York. (Chapter 9)

1966 – DMT association is founded in the United States. (Chapter 7)

1966 – Rudolf von Laban writes *Choreutics*. (Chapter 9)

1968 – Merce Cunningham creates *RainForest*. (Chapter 5)

1968 – Martin Luther King Jr. is assassinated. (Chapter 5)

1968 – The Tet Offensive, orchestrated by Ho Chi Minh and leaders in Hanoi, is launched in Vietnam. (Chapter 5)

1969 – Arthur Mitchell and Karel Shook found the Dance Theatre of Harlem. (Chapter 4)

1970–2010 – Many dance films, often about self-expression, are made with notable advances in dialog and storytelling. (Chapter 8)

Early 1970s – Dance Theatre of Harlem starts wearing flesh-tone tights. (Chapter 4)

1970s – Bonnie Bainbridge Cohen develops the Body-Mind Centering (BMC) school. (Chapter 7)

1970s – DMT provides curricular training in colleges in the United States. (Chapter 7)

1970s–1980s – In New York City, breaking emerges as a popular dance form. On the West Coast, popping, locking, and whaacking develop. By the 1980s, these aesthetics merge to become known as hip hop dance. Breaking is featured in the 1984 Summer Olympics Opening Ceremony in Los Angeles. (Chapter 3)

1972 – "Trail of Broken Treaties" march happens to Washington, D.C. and the subsequent occupation of the Bureau of Indian Affairs. (Chapter 1)

1972 – Fosse creates *Cabaret*. (Chapter 8)

1973 – *Ashani Sanket* puts India on the world map as a cinema powerhouse. (Chapter 8)

1973 – Wounded Knee Occupation, also referred to as a "Ghost Dance," occurs. (Chapter 1)

1975 – Lydia Abarca became the first Black ballerina to appear on the cover of *Dance Magazine*. (Chapter 4)

1978 – American Indian Religious Freedom Act ends previously banned Native dance. (Chapter 1)

1980s – DMT provides curricular training in colleges in England and Australasia. (Chapter 7)

1980s – VNS (Very Nervous System) is created. (Chapter 9)

1980s–2000s – Hip hop, Michael Jackson's choreography, and other Africanist-based dance forms spread across the globe, aided by MTV and other means of dissemination. (Chapter 3)

1982 – Debra Austin became the first Black principal dancer promoted at Pennsylvania Ballet. (Chapter 4)

1990 – Lauren Anderson became the first Black principal dancer at Houston Ballet and continued the racialized declaration of wearing flesh-tone tights. (Chapter 4)

1990 – Israeli dance artist Ohad Naharin becomes the artistic director of the Batsheva Dance Company and develops Gaga. (Chapter 7)

1990–1999 – LifeForms (later DanceForms) is developed and used. (Chapter 9)

1990s – The term "dance technology" started to be used. (Chapter 9)

1992 – April 11 – Seo Tajji and Boys performed "Nan Arayo (I Know)" on a South Korean talent show, marking the beginning of K-pop. (Chapter 8)

2000s–2020s – Greater acknowledgment of the Africanist roots of dance innovations in the Americas across all sectors of dance – concert dance, Broadway dance, popular entertainment, and social dance. Debates about cultural appropriation and the stealing of Black dances increase with the proliferation of social media platforms such as YouTube and TikTok that make such dances go "viral." (Chapter 3)

2005 – February 14 – YouTube is launched. (Chapter 10)

2006 – *Glow* is performed. (Chapter 9)

2006 – *Memoirs of Active Service* is choreographed. (Chapter 5)

2010 – October 6 – Instagram is launched. (Chapter 10)

2014 – A hologram of Michael Jackson is screened at the Billboard Music Awards stage. (Chapter 10)

2015 – Misty Copeland becomes the first Black principal dancer at ABT on their 75th Anniversary. (Chapter 4).

2017 – *Through You* is released. (Chapter 10)

2019 – Emovere, *Fragile Intersections* is performed. (Chapter 9)

2019 – WhoLoDancE project begins. (Chapter 10)

2020 – March – COVID-19 prompts series of lockdowns. (Chapter 10)

# Glossary

**Afrocubanismo movement** – this refers to the artistic movement in Cuba in the 1920s and 1930s in which black culture became accepted.

**Apart dancing** – apart dancing is a feature of West African dance in which individuals dance separately, or even together, but do not touch.

**Apollonian** – this term refers to the rational aspect of human nature.

**Artificial Intelligence** – a term that refers to computer systems built to mimic human intelligence.

**Centrifugal movement** – this term explains movement that relies on the outward force that is felt as a dancer rotates.

**Co-regulation** – a process that relies on the concept that the nervous system of one person influences that of another.

**Courtiers** – this term refers to a companion or advisor to the royalty in a court.

**Cyberspace** – this term refers to the space between two or more computer systems.

**Dhol** – this is a double-sided barrel drum used in India.

**Expressionism** – an artistic style that depicts a subjective experience.

**Greenwich Village Follies** – a multi-act musical production that performed from 1919–1927.

**Harlem Renaissance** – a period of African American cultural and intellectual activity that took place in Harlem, New York City in the 20s and 30s.

**Highbrow and lowbrow art** – these terms are used to describe art that is considered to be either sophisticated or of low entertainment value.

**Holistic** – emphasizing the interconnectedness of all the parts of something.

**Hologram** – this technology allows for a picture to be taken then presented in three dimensions.

**I-Ching** – translated as "The Book of Changes," this book is a classic Taoist text that discusses divination.

**Interdisciplinary** – a term that denotes drawing from multiple disciplines.

**Kinetoscope** – a device used to watch early motion pictures.

**Ladja** – the ladja is a sacred dance from Martinique.

**Livestreaming** – this technology allows for something to be recorded and broadcasted at the same time.

**Montage** – a film technique that brings together selections of a film to form a sequence.

**Proscenium stage** – a stage with an arch that separates the stage from the audience.

**Sagittal** – this adjective refers to the suture at the top of the skull that divides the body into left and right.

**Settler colonialism** – a form of colonialism in which colonists attempt to replace Native populations with their new society.

**Sovereignty** – authority over a place.

**Survivance** – a term coined by Gerald Vizenor, who defines it as "an active sense of presence, the continuance of native stories, not a mere reaction, or a survivable name. Native survivance stories are renunciations of dominance, tragedy and victimry."

**Systemic racism** – a term to describe racism that is written into institutions and policies.

**Tawaif** – an entertainer in the Mughal era.

**The *grouillère*** – a traditional Haitian dance.

**The Middle Passage** – this term refers to the forced passage from Africa to the Americas in the Atlantic slave trade.

**Transdisciplinary** – a term that denotes integrating multiple disciplines.

**Tulsa Race Riots** – now called the Tulsa Race Massacre, this term refers to the violent destruction of and murders in the Greenwood District, a predominantely black neighborhood, after the arrest of Dick Rowland.

**Vaudeville** – a variety-show style entertainment popular in the early 20th century.

**Yellow Peril** – a term used to describe European and American racist "fears" of Asia.

**Zoom** – this software is a video calling platform.

**Zoroastrianism** – an Iranian, pre-Islamic religion.

# Further Viewing and Reading

*A Ballerina's Tale Documentary A Ballerina's Tale* provides a behind-the-scenes of Misty Copeland and the triumphs and struggles that she and dancers before her experience as Black women in ballet.

Armor, John and Wright, Peter. *Manzanar* with photos by Ansel Adams, New York: Times Books, 1988. This book gives insights into life at the Japanese American Internment Camp, *Manzanar*. Through documented stories and photographs of the camp and its inhabitants, the injustice faced by Japanese Americans under Executive Order 9066 is revealed. This publication is especially useful in understanding the reality of Michio Itō's circumstance from 1941–1943.

Au, Susan. "Ballet and Modern Dance." *ASSESSMENT* 1, no. 2 (1974): 3. *Ballet and Modern Dance* provides a historical guide to ballet and modern dance from Medici to Manhattan, New York. Au provides a foundation in which she highlights significant historical moments and people throughout the dance world.

Ballantyne, Tony. *Between Colonialism and Diaspora: Sikh Cultural Formations in an Imperial World.* Durham: Duke University Press, 2006. Ballantyne traces the remarkable journey of a village harvest dance that became a transnational symbol of Sikh identity and a powerful testimony of resilience.

Billman, Larry. Film *Choreographers and Dance Directors: An Illustrated Biographical Encyclopedia.* Jefferson, NC: McFarland and Company: 1997. This encyclopedic text features nearly 1,000 film dance choreographers and dance directors as well as the 3,500 films to which they contributed choreography and dance direction. Readers can efficiently learn about the work of these artists individually and also piece together a more comprehensive view of the evolution of this art form from the tail end of the 19th century to the end of the 20th.

Birringer, J., (ed). 2002. "Dance and Digital Media." Special issue prepared and edited for *Performing Arts Journal* 70, introduction, pp. 84–93. This paper proposes a classification on the new aesthetics of interactivity in dance, describing different types of dance interaction, depending on the technical context and the artistic challenges when working with real-time processing.

*Black Ballerina Documentary* https://blackballerinadocumentary.org.

*Black Ballerina* shares stories of Black women of several generations who became ballerinas. They share their racialized experiences and how they continue to challenge the racial stereotypes used to exclude Black women from ballet.

Bleeker, Maaike. *Transmission in Motion: The Technologizing of Dance.* 1st Edition. ISBN 9781138189447. October 4, 2016 by Routledge. When we discuss motion, more specifically dance, there is a personalization and realism that we expect. There is a need to feel and see things from a human perspective that we may not expect to be attainable through technology. However, *Transmission in Motion: The Technologizing of Dance* strives to show the mutual connection between various technologies, from a conventional standpoint to newer avenues, and how those can be used to better understand dance movement.

Branningham, Erin. *Dancefilm: Choreography and the Moving Image.* London: Oxford University Press: 2011. Branningham's text offers both historical context and artistic analysis of choreographic work on film – highlighting the most influential events as well as painting a picture of the evolution of dance on film more broadly. The text also merges choreographic theory and film theory, the latter being a field of creative study that dancers and dance enthusiasts might not know as much of but could benefit from learning about.

Brave Bird, Mary, and Richard Erdoes. *Lakota Woman.* New York: Grove Press, 1990. Narrated from the perspective of Mary Brave Bird, a Sicangu Lakota woman, this memoir provides further insight into how Lakota and other Native peoples have navigated and/or thwarted the structures of U.S. settler colonialism, including patriarchy. In particular, the text details Brave Bird's participation in the American Indian Movement, including her involvement in the 1972 Trail of Broken Treaties and the 1973 Indian Occupation at Wounded Knee.

Browner, Tara. *Heartbeat of the People: Music and Dance of the Northern Pow-Wow.* Champaign: University of Illinois Press, 2002. In this influential book, Tara Browner (Choctaw), an ethnomusicologist and Jingle Dress Dancer, draws on her own experiences as well as interviews with other pow-wow practitioners to delineate the history and politics of the Northern pow-wow of the Northern Plains and Great Lakes. The text contextualizes in detail a variety of tribally-specific and pan-Native American practices, including the Jingle Dress Dance, Omaha Dance, songs, and regalia, to demonstrate the capacities of pow-wow to produce tribal affiliation.

Caldwell, Helen. *Michio Ito: The Dancer and His Dances.* Los Angeles: The University of California Press, 1977. This book traces the beginnings of Itō's career in Europe, its expansion in New York, and finally to its climax in California before his repatriation in 1942. Of especial interest are the historic photos of Itō's repertoire and his dance technique.

Chakravorty, Pallabi. *Bells of Change: Kathak Dance, Women, and Modernity in India.* Kolkata: Seagull Books, 2008. The author, a South Asian feminist with a doctorate in anthropology, offers a fresh investigation into the origins and development of Kathak that highlights the marginalized voices of women.

Chatterjea, Ananya. *Heat and Alterity in Contemporary Dance.* Palgrave Macmillan, 2020. Chatterjea exposes the systemic exclusions embedded in the construction of categories like "contemporary dance" and analyzes the work of Germaine Acogny, Sardono Kusumo, Nora Chipaumire, Rulan Tangen, Lemi Ponifasio, Camille Brown, Prumsodun Ok, and Alice Sheppard.

Clemmens, Michael. *Embodied Relational Gestalt: Theories and Applications.* Taylor & Francis, 2019. The eclectic group of authors and subjects in this book are a testament to the philosophical foundation of Gestalt Therapy, achieving a multiplicity of individual understandings within a collective whole. The reader will have a broad perspective of how Gestalt Therapy can guide a person into an embodied relational experience.

Cohen, Bonnie Bainbridge. *Sensing, Feeling, and Action: The Experiential Anatomy of Body-Mind Centering.* First Paperback Edition. Northampton, MA: Contact Editions, 1994. This book is a collection of articles and writings written by Bonnie Bainbridge Cohen on essential themes in Body-Mind Centering (BMC) education. Although BMC has evolved since these articles were written, the open gaps are inviting and may inspire students' own embodied research.

Croft, Clare. *Dancers as Diplomats: American Choreography in Cultural Exchange.* Oxford: Oxford University Press, 2015. Croft describes touring programs created by the State Department of the United States and the networks of institutional support that promoted the work of certain choreographers and dance companies.

Daniel, Yvonne. *Dancing Wisdom: Embodied Knowledge in Haitian Vodou, Cuban Yoruba, and Bahian Candomblé.* Urbana: University of Illinois, 2005. *Dancing Wisdom* argues that dance is a central component of African diasporic religious practices in the circum-Caribbean. She analyzes the aesthetic and philosophical components of Vodou, Yoruba, and Candomblé through ethnographic fieldwork and combines that with theoretical work on African diasporic religions. By investigating three different forms, she showcases distinctions as well as similarities.

DeFrantz, Thomas F. and Anita Gonzalez, eds. *Black Performance Theory.* Durham, NC: Duke University Press, 2014. This book assembles many of the most important scholars of Black Dance, Theatre, and Performance Studies. The authors tackle globalization, the digital information revolution, new expressions of gender and sexuality, challenges to essentialized identity categories, and the turn to diaspora as a "meta-discourse" in their analyses of Black performance. DeFrantz and

Gonzalez's introduction, which provides a genealogy of how generations of scholars have addressed questions about Blackness in relation to performance, is particularly useful.

Dixon, S. 2007. *Digital Performance – A History of New Media in Theater, Dance, Performance, Art, and Installation.* The MIT Press. An excellent book that presents the historical roots, key practitioners, and artistic, theoretical, and technological trends in the incorporation of new media into the performing arts. Steve Dixon traces the evolution of these practices, presents detailed accounts of key practitioners and performances, and analyzes the theoretical, artistic, and technological contexts of this form of new media art.

Eddy, Martha. *Mindful Movement: The Evolution of the Somatic Arts and Conscious Action.* Intellect Books, 2016. Martha Eddy edits and contributes an essential and comprehensive introduction of the history and theories of mindful movement practices. This book also describes the evolution of the field of mindful movement studies from an educational paradigm into a therapeutic one.

Evans, Mark and Mary Fogarty. *Movies, Moves and Music: The Sonic World of Dance Films.* Sheffield, UK: Equinox Publishing, 2016. This text investigates the intersection of music and movement in the medium of film, from the post-War period to the present – historically, globally, socioculturally, and creatively. Pop culture phenomena such as Bollywood, as well as stylistic instances of dancers creating sound through their performance (such as in Irish dance, Flamenco, and Krumping), are described.

Foster, Susan Leigh. "Choreographies and Choreographers," in *Worlding Dance: Studies in International Performance.* New York: Palgrave Macmillan, 2009. This book chapter explores the "othering" and "forgetting" of Michio Itō due to the labeling of him as an international artist which came in conflict with U.S. nationalism. This chapter considers the effects of the racialization of Itō's migration story on his career and legacy.

Gaiser, Carrie. "Caught Dancing: Hybridity, Stability, and Subversion in Dance Theatre of Harlem's Creole 'Giselle'." *Theatre Journal* (2006): 269–289. "Caught Dancing: Hybridity, Stability, and Subversion in Dance Theatre of Harlem's Creole 'Giselle' examines Dance Theatre of Harlem's production of *Creole Giselle* and elaborates on the conjunction of Black dancing bodies and European classical ballet style techniques. This article provides additional information on racial and cultural negotiations within ballet.

Genne, Beth. *Dance Me a Song: Astaire, Balanchine, Kelly, and the American Film Musical.* London: Oxford University Press, 2018. Genne's text explores the work of these three iconic dance artists and choreographers, and how it both drew from, and came to shape, American pop culture – reflecting American values of pluralism, multiplicity, and the possibility of a better life for any person. Genne also describes how technological advancements and innovations in the craft of directing in conjunction with these artists' works pushed dance on film forward, to ultimately have that culture-sharing effect.

Gottschild, Brenda Dixon. *Digging the Africanist Presence in American Performance: Dance and Other Contexts*. Westport: Greenwood Press, 1996. Dr Gottschild's book transformed dance studies by challenging the perceived whiteness of concert dance genres such as ballet, modern, and postmodern dance. Terms that she coins in this book, such as "invisibilization" and "Africanist," have become standard in analyzing how dance operates in the United States. Gottschild highlights the tremendous influence of Africanist aesthetics on dance and choreography in the United States, and reveals how and why these influences are often undocumented or misattributed.

Gottschild, Brenda. *The black dancing body: A geography from coon to cool*. Springer, 2016. *The black dancing body* provides a chronological map of Black bodies throughout a variety of different dance genres. Gottschild addresses the influence and importance of Black bodies throughout dance history which has historically been omitted from many dance history literatures.

Hall, Stuart. "The West and the Rest: Discourse and Power," in *The Formations of Modernity*. Cambridge: The Open University, 1992. Hall examines how discourses, such as "the West" or "Western civilization," are produced and maintained to assert power and to delimit which people and cultures have access to that power, as well as which do not.

Hansen, Valerie. *The Silk Road: A New History*. Oxford: Oxford University Press, 2012. This innovative approach uses archeological evidence to replace the romanticized Silk Road with a reality evidenced by physical objects that tell cultural, social, and economic stories of cross-cultural exchange. Hansen focuses on seven important trade centers, illustrating her findings with vivid color plates.

Hokowhitu, Brendan. "Haka: Colonized Physicality, Body-Logic, and Embodied Sovereignty," in *Performing Indigeneity: Global Histories and Contemporary Experiences*. Edited by H. Glenn Penny and Laura R. Graham, 273–304. Lincoln: University of Nebraska Press, 2014. This article by a Māori scholar discusses how colonizers in New Zealand have appropriated, leveraged, and (mis)represented haka for settler colonial and capitalist purposes while Māori peoples have danced the haka for the purposes of enacting self-representation/sovereignty. Given that discourses have frequently relegated Indigenous peoples and practices to the past, the author posits that doing the haka is a way of enacting sovereignty in the "immediate" present and forwarding Māori epistemologies specifically on the level of the body, which challenges Cartesian dualism.

Jaimovich, J. and Morand, F. (2019). "Shaping the Biology of Emotion: Emovere, an Interactive Performance." *International Journal of Performance Arts and Digital Media*, 15:1, 35–52, doi:10.1080/14794713.2018.1563 354. This paper presents a detailed example of the artistic creation and research work of an interactive dance and sound performance with bio-sensors. *Emovere* (2015) is based on the biology of emotion in association with physiological signals and the induction of emotional states from corporeal patterns.

Johnson, Don. Bone, Breath & Gesture: Practices of Embodiment. North Atlantic Books, 1995. Don Johnson compiles original writings of pio-neers in mindful movement dance classes, somatics, dance/movement therapy, and body psychotherapy. This book collection of essays is a must-have for mindful movers interested in the original writings and the legacy that came before them.

Lewin, Yaël Tamar, and Janet Collins. *Night's dancer: the life of Janet Collins*. Wesleyan University Press, 2011. *Night's dancer: the life of Janet Collins* is a biography about Janet Collins and how she broke barriers as the first Black woman to be a prima ballerina. This book provides a depth insight into the racialized experience of Janet Collins in ballet.

Mitoma, Judy. *Envisioning Dance on Film and Video*. London: Routledge Publishing, 2003. Through the voices of those working in the field, including choreographers, cinematographers, and critics, this work takes a deep dive into the intersection of dance and film. Readers therein can gain a multidisciplinary, multi-perspective look into dance on film, from those who know it in a deep, experiential way.

Pallaro, Patrizia. *Authentic Movement: Essays by Mary Starks Whitehouse, Janet Adler and Joan Chodorow*. Jessica Kingsley Publishers, 1999. Patrizia Pallaro compiles in one place eight chapters of original writings by the founder of Authentic Movement (Mary Starks Whitehouse) and thir-teen chapters by her main students (Janet Adler and Joan Chodorow), who have advanced the studies to a well-known Dance/Movement Therapy practice. These original writings illuminate the context in the development of the practice, its analytical theoretical foundation, and the discoveries made in the beginning stages of teaching the nuances of Authentic Movement.

Raheja, Michelle. "Visual Sovereignty." In *Native Studies Keywords*. Edited by Andrea Smith, Michelle Raheja, Stephanie Nohelani Teves, 25–34. Tucson: University of Arizona Press, 2015. In this article, Michelle Raheja discusses the complex meanings of sovereignty – a central concept in Indigenous studies – in Native American/First Nations/ Indigenous contexts. Although until recently, scholars have primarily written about sovereignty in the legal realm and social sciences and in ways that are recognizable to the settler state, the author emphasizes that broader and Native-centered understandings of sovereignty that often value creative and embodied forms of knowledge – such as Indigenous dance – are critical.

Rosenberg, Douglas. *Screendance: Inscribing the Ephemeral Image.* New York: Oxford University Press, 2012. Rosenberg's text, both a history and a critical analysis, takes a rigorous and academic look at film dance. Rosenberg calls upon analytic frames, from the psycho-analytic to the feminist to the literary, to probe deeper into meaningful intersections within dance on film – dancer and audience member, dancer and director, dancer (or other subject) and the camera.

Ross, Janice. *Moving Lessons: Margaret H'Doubler and the Beginning of Dance in American Education.* Madison: University of Wisconsin Press, 2000. Ross traces the development of the first dance degree program in the United States, created by Margaret H'Doubler at the University of Wisconsin-Madison.

Shea Murphy, Jacqueline. *The People Have Never Stopped Dancing: Native American Modern Dance Histories.* Minneapolis: University of Minnesota Press, 2007. Shea Murphy provides both a historical and theoretical account of the importance of Native dance and amplifies the importance of dance's transformative abilities. This innovative and comprehensive text presents the first book-length study of the history and politics of contemporary Native American dance. Some of what the author illuminates includes: how Native peoples have navigated U.S. prohibitions surrounding Indigenous movement modes; how "pioneering," non-Native, modern dance choreographers have appropriated Native dance forms and drawn on, and profited from, their (mis)conceptions about "Indianness"; the emergence of Aboriginal and Native American stage dance in the 1960s and 1970s; and the unique works of Indigenous choreographers today, which may also include commonalities among them, such as thematic concerns with the connections between past and present as well as human and more-than-human kin.

Sparshott, Francis. "The Future of Dance Aesthetics." *The Journal of Aesthetics and Art Criticism* 51, no. 2 (1993): 227–234. doi:10.2307/431389. Aesthetics plays a pivotal role in how we perceive things around us. This pertains to many aspects of life whether scientific, philosophical, etc. The arts are no different when it comes to aesthetics, which begs the question of how the subject of aesthetics could coincide with technology and how it relates to the future of where dance will go.

Tharp, T. "On Technology and Dance." *Encyclopedia Britannica*, July 22, 2005. www.britannica.com/topic/technology-and-dance-1082484. How technology can contribute to dance and the way we view dance education and performance is a question with many possible answers. Tharp dives into the ways which we have become accustomed to receiving dance performance while highlighting how technology elevates that experience.

Walker, Margaret E. *India's Kathak Dance in Historical Perspective*. Farnham, England: Ashgate, 2014. The author investigates the accepted origin stories of Kathak to reveal a complex and fascinating history of a dance form that endured colonialism and post-colonial backlash to become global performance art.

Warren, Larry. *Lester Horton: Modern Dance Pioneer*. New York: Marcel Dekker, Inc., 1977. This is a comprehensive biography of Lester Horton, the protégé of Michio Itō and the mentor of Alvin Ailey. This book allows the reader to understand the historical impact of Itō's legacy on multiple generations of dancer in America.

Wechsler, R., "Artistic Considerations in the Use of Motion Tracking with Live Performers: A Practical Guide," in *Performance and Technology: Practices of Virtual Embodiment and Interactivity* edited by Susan Broadhurst and Josephine Machon, Palgrave Macmillian, 2006. This specific chapter focuses on the practical uses and the artistic implications of motion tracking, describing key concepts as interaction, real time, and mapping, as well as an analysis of one of the iconic softwares for movement interactivity: Eyecon.

Welsh, Kariamu, Esailama G.A. Diouf, and Yvonne Daniel, eds. *Hot Feet and Social Change: African Dance and Diaspora Communities*. Urbana: University of Illinois Press, 2019. This recent book, edited by some of the most important scholars in African diasporic dance studies, showcases the breadth and richness of African dance in the Americas, particularly the United States. Far from viewing African influence as something of the pre-modern past, these authors demonstrate how West, Central, and South African dancers, musicians, and choreographers have influenced dance in the United States in the 20th and 21st centuries.

Witbeck, Quisqueya G. "Breaking Boundaries: Bhangra as a Mechanism for Identity Formation and Sociopolitical Refuge Among South Asian American Youths." ProQuest Dissertations Publishing, 2018. This dissertation reveals the profound and positive impact of a folk dance on minority youth in their search for identity.

Wong, Yutian. *Choreographing Asian America*. Middleton: Wesleyan University Press, 2010. Wong analyzes relationships between Asian America and American dance history, paying close attention to the intertwining of representations, identities, and stereotypes.

# Index

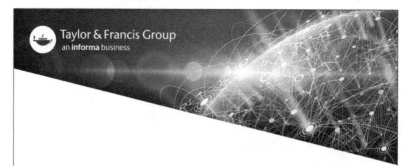